T0257588

Theory and Advanced Researches in Orthodontics

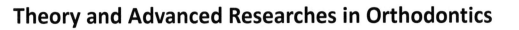

Theory and Advanced Researches in Orthodontics

Edited by **Kaley Ann**

FOSTER
A C A D E M I C S

New Jersey

Published by Foster Academics,
61 Van Reypen Street,
Jersey City, NJ 07306, USA
www.fosteracademics.com

Theory and Advanced Researches in Orthodontics
Edited by Kaley Ann

International Standard Book Number: 978-1-63242-396-2 (Hardback)

Contents

; unique book which encompasses the most up-to-date
pleased to get this opportunity of editing the work of
ave also written papers in this field and researched the
the progress of the discipline. I have tried to unify my
dwarts from every corner of the world, to produce a text
ers but also facilitates the growth of the field.

s and advanced work contributed by several academic and
sses topics like epidemiological & prevention and growth &
an analysis of the most important information, studies the
perts and their efforts to educate readers with quality content
cia   tions and rising trends in orthodontics. The book is intended for both
dents as   practitioners associated with the field of orthodontics. It will assist them
acquiring valuable and authentic knowledge and excellent clinical skills.

ally, I would like to thank all the contributing authors for their valuable time and
tributions. This book would not have been possible without their efforts. I would also
e to thank my friends and family for their constant support.

Editor

Preface

I am honored to present to you this unique book which encompasses the most up-to-date data in the field. I was extremely pleased to get this opportunity of editing the work of experts from across the globe. I have also written papers in this field and researched the various aspects revolving around the progress of the discipline. I have tried to unify my knowledge along with that of stalwarts from every corner of the world, to produce a text which not only benefits the readers but also facilitates the growth of the field.

This book provides the theories and advanced work contributed by several academic and research veterans. It encompasses topics like epidemiological & prevention and growth & genetic. The sections present an analysis of the most important information, studies the knowledge illustrated by experts and their efforts to educate readers with quality content elucidating novel directions and rising trends in orthodontics. The book is intended for both students as well as practitioners associated with the field of orthodontics. It will assist them in acquiring valuable and authentic knowledge and excellent clinical skills.

Finally, I would like to thank all the contributing authors for their valuable time and contributions. This book would not have been possible without their efforts. I would also like to thank my friends and family for their constant support.

Editor

Part 1

Epidemiology and Prevention

Orthodontic Treatment Need: An Epidemiological Approach

Carlos Bellot-Arcís, José María Montiel-Company and
José Manuel Almerich-Silla
Stomatology Department, University of Valencia
Spain

1. Introduction

The main aim of orthodontic treatment is to correct malocclusion, in order, whenever possible, to achieve functionally appropriate occlusion and optimum dental and facial aesthetics. To understand what malocclusion is, first we need to define its antonyms, in other words, what is meant by normal occlusion and ideal occlusion. Normal occlusion can be said to be that which meets certain predefined standards.

Edward Hartley Angle (1899) took the first permanent molars as the reference point and established the precise relations between the two dental arches that could be considered "norm-occlusion". "Normal occlusion" was thus defined as a concrete goal that the orthodontist should aim for in order to achieve a structural, functional and aesthetic norm (Canut, 1988). Since Angle's days, normal occlusion and ideal occlusion have been treated as synonyms in orthodontics, giving rise to both semantic and treatment difficulties. Nevertheless, from the statistical point of view the term "normal" implies a certain variation around the mean, while "ideal" implies a concept of perfection as the hypothetical aim (Bravo, 2003).

The occlusal norms that all orthodontists, over many years of professional practice, had borne in mind when deciding their clinical objectives were set out by Andrews (1972) in an article describing the six keys to normal occlusion. He later changed the adjective "normal" occlusion to "optimal" occlusion, arguing that he had used the word "normal" in the sense of optimal or ideal, as was often the case in the 1970s, and that normal occlusion was more correctly called "non-optimal occlusion".

"Orthodontic treatment need" can be defined as the degree to which a person needs orthodontic treatment because of certain features of his or her malocclusion, the functional, dental health or aesthetic impairment it occasions and the negative psychological and social repercussions to which it gives rise.

Throughout the history of orthodontics, there have been authors who have considered that malocclusion can lead to other problems, such as functional problems, temporomandibular dysfunction, and a greater propensity to trauma, caries, or periodontal disease. However, nowadays it is not so evident that these processes or diseases constitute indications for orthodontic treatment. Generally speaking, the psychological and social implications of poor dentofacial aesthetics can be more serious than the biological problems, and in clinical trials, strong correlations have been found between dental aesthetics, treatment need and the severity of the malocclusion (Lewis et al., 1982). Hamdam (2004) concluded that 40% of the patients who underwent orthodontic treatment had been the butt of jokes because of their teeth. However, there was no association between the degree of orthodontic treatment need measured by an objective index (IOTN DHC) and the need perceived by the patients. Kiekens et al. (2006) concluded that what the patients hope for from orthodontic treatment is an improvement in their dentofacial aesthetics and, as a result, greater social acceptance and higher self-esteem. Because of this, in recent decades orthodontists have been increasingly directing their treatments towards improving facial aesthetics.

Strictly speaking, malocclusion is not an illness but an occlusal relationship that lies within the bounds of all the possible occlusal relationships. Deciding the exact point at which a specific malocclusion should be treated remains an open question among orthodontists and the subject of considerable debate in the literature, as owing to its nature, reaching a general consensus is proving really complicated.

The WHO (World Health Organization) defines health as "a state of complete physical, mental and social well-being and not merely the absence of disease or infirmity". Consequently, a person cannot be considered completely healthy if a malocclusion prevents him or her from attaining this state of complete well-being, whether for physical (functional impairment) or psycho-social reasons (serious impairment of self-esteem or dentofacial aesthetics).

Disease does not always entail the absence of well-being, and even when well-being is absent this depends to a large extent on the patient's psychological state and personal and cultural principles and values. While clinical indices are concerned to measure the "disease", a purely biological concept, as objectively as possible, the indices that attempt to measure and determine "health" are very subjective, as health is a more psychological or sociological concept (Bernabé & Flores-Mir, 2006).

It should be emphasized that there is a lack of agreement on what is or is not considered malocclusion, and even greater disagreement when determining the orthodontic treatment need. However, enormous progress in this direction has been made in recent years, with important areas of consensus being reached among the specialists concerning specific situations in which orthodontic treatment should be recommended. The rapid development of indices to measure malocclusion and orthodontic treatment need have unquestionably contributed to these advances.

2. Using indices to measure malocclusion

2.1 Definition of "index"

Indices are quantitative assessment tools, employing continuous or numbered scales of malocclusion for epidemiological purposes and for a number of administrative applications.

An orthodontic treatment need index assigns a specific score to each malocclusion feature according to that feature's relative contribution to the overall severity of the malocclusion.

Each occlusal feature measured by a particular index is assigned a quantitative value or specific weight based on personal clinical concepts, consensus among specialists, reviews of the literature, social and administrative needs or scientific studies designed specifically for this purpose, hence the great variety of very different indices for recording malocclusion, which can have many uses.

Occlusal indices decide the need for treatment from the point of view of the orthodontist but tend to ignore the patients' own perceptions of their malocclusion and the repercussions it has in their daily lives, not only from a functional point of view but also on their looks, which undoubtedly have an effect on their social relationships. The traditional indices do not give any type of information on how the malocclusion affects the patients' lives from the psychosocial or functional point of view. These aspects seem to have become particularly important in recent years (Kok et al., 2004).

2.2 History, evolution, classification and properties of treatment need indices

Attempts to classify dentofacial disharmony date back to the beginning of the 19th century, to authors such as Joseph Fox (1776-1816), Christophe François Delabarre (1784-1862), Jean Nicolas Marjolin (1780-1850), Friedrich Christoph Kneisel (1797-1847) or Georg Carabelli (1787-1842). It was not until 1899, however, that Edward Hartley Angle (1855-1930) developed a clear, simple, practical classification that became universally accepted and used. Nonetheless, this index has evident limitations from the epidemiological point of view.

Angle's classification has been followed by many others. That of Lischer (1912) was similar but introduced the terms neutrocclusion (Angle Class I), mesiocclusion (Angle Class III) and distocclusion (Angle Class II). Simon (1922) proposed a classification that sets out the relation between the dental arches by reference to the three anatomical planes, based on different points on the skull. Dewey and Anderson (1942) published a book in which they extended Angle's classification to include five types of Class I malocclusion and three types of Class III malocclusion, known as the Dewey-Anderson Modification. The classification of Ackerman and Proffit (1969) was intended to overcome Angle's main weaknesses; however, it is more of a diagnostic procedure for listing the problems in each case of malocclusion in order to assist the clinician in drawing up a treatment plan.

All the methods described so far are qualitative and serve to describe and classify a patient's malocclusion. However, countries that have health services which offer orthodontic treatment have developed and applied a series of quantitative methods (malocclusion indices) to detect the severity and treatment need of each case, in an attempt to define the priority of some cases over others objectively and thus rationalize their public expenditure.

Tang and Wei (1993) reviewed the literature and summarized the evolution of methods for recording malocclusion in recent decades. They concluded that the trend in both qualitative and quantitative methods has changed, as initially researchers did not define the signs of malocclusion before recording them, chose the variables arbitrarily and recorded the data according to a criterion of all or nothing. This has now changed and a study of the progress in occlusal recording methods shows that they are increasingly accurate, reliable and scientifically-based, and consequently their detection of the problems possesses greater validity.

According to Richmond et al. (1997), an orthodontic index should consist of a numerical scale obtained by considering specific features of the malocclusion, making it possible to determine certain parameters such as treatment need or the severity of malocclusion in an objective way.

In 1966 the World Health Organization (WHO) defined the three characteristics that an index should possess: reliability, validity and validity over time.

There is wide agreement that an orthodontic treatment need index should possess the following characteristics·

- **Validity:** an index is said to be valid if it measures what it aims to measure. If a problem exists, it must detect it exactly and without error. In other words, it must identify the patients with the most detrimental malocclusions or those who would most benefit from treatment.
- **Objectivity:** the index design must attempt as far as possible to exclude examiner subjectivity.
- **Reliability (accuracy or reproducibility):** this is the degree of match between the results obtained when an index is applied to the same sample by different examiners or by the same examiner on different occasions.
- **Simplicity:** it must be able to be used by non-specialists. It must be capable of distinguishing between benign malocclusions that do not require treatment and more serious cases that need to be treated by a specialist.
- **Flexibility:** an index must be easily modified over time in the light of new research, discoveries or considerations.
- **Appropriate assessment of the aesthetic component of the malocclusion.**

Prahl-Andersen (1978) described the features that in his opinion an orthodontic treatment need index should possess. He emphasized that an index should not establish treatment priorities solely on the basis of the severity of the malocclusion and the functional problems that it could entail. It should also assess the degree to which the malocclusion occasions aesthetic impairment. In the medical field, a person's health should be judged on three criteria: objective signs (the orthodontist's diagnosis), subjective symptoms (the patient must recognize the problem) and social sufficiency (social attitudes).

Shaw et al. (1995) highlighted the following uses of the indices:

- Classifying, planning and promoting treatment standards.
- Assisting dentists and pediatric dentists to identify patients with orthodontic treatment need.
- Identifying patient prognoses and obtaining the patients' informed consent, informing them of the risks and treatment stability in both severe and borderline cases.
- Assessing the difficulty of the treatment that a particular patient must follow.
- Assessing the results of the treatment.

Throughout the history of orthodontics, indices have been developed to record malocclusions. Abdullah and Rock (2001) considered that most of them must have been developed with the following aims:

- To classify malocclusions in order to allow and facilitate communication between professionals.
- To compile a database to facilitate epidemiological studies.
- To classify cases according to the complexity of their treatment.
- To determine treatment needs and priorities.
- To identify the aesthetic aspects that affect treatment need.

It must not be forgotten that orthodontic treatment need indices, or at least most of them, are designed to determine treatment priority, in other words, to choose the potential patients who will most benefit from orthodontic treatment in a particular health service system.

In Europe, occlusal indices to estimate treatment need have been being used successfully since the end of the 1980s. The indices employed have generally been those developed by european authors but there has been no unanimity as regards which method to employ.

The controversy that surrounds orthodontic treatment need indices is such that in the United States, in 1969 the American Orthodontic Society adopted and recommended the *Salzmann Index* for estimating the treatment needs of the population but withdrew its recommendation in 1985 and currently does not recognize any index as more suitable than any other for this purpose (Parker, 1998).

Many very different indices have been developed to classify and group malocclusions according to severity or level of treatment need.

3. Principal treatment need indices

The *Malalignment Index* was developed by Van Kirk (1959) because he considered that there was no way of classifying patients objectively according to their tooth or bone malalignment. In this index, each tooth is given a score between 0 and 2 depending on its degree of rotation or displacement compared to the ideal position in the dental arch.

The state of New York started its Dental Rehabilitation Program in 1945 and one of the main problems was to select the patients who would receive orthodontic treatment. As a result, Draker (1960) developed and published *Handicapping Labio-lingual Deviation* (HLD) with the aim of determining orthodontic treatment need. This index assesses 7 criteria (displacement, crowding, overjet, increased overbite, open bite, anterior crossbite and ectopic eruptions) exclusively in the anterior sector, and also takes malformations into account. It can be applied both to models and to examinations of the mouth. When the scores for all the criteria total over 13, the subject is considered to present a physical malocclusion that needs treatment.

The *Treatment Priority Index* (TPI) was developed by Grainger (1967). This index is based on an assessment of ten occlusal features measured in a representative sample of 375 children of 12 years of age, of Anglo-Saxon origin, all without previous orthodontic treatment. The children were examined directly by orthodontic specialists. The patient is considered to need treatment when the scores for the ten occlusal features total over 4.5. A further eleventh feature is only considered in special cases (cleft palate or dysmorphism caused by traumatic injury) in which treatment is a priority. TPI has been used in many studies and although the results have not always been regular, it has proved to give high intra-examiner and inter-examiner reproducibility and reasonably good validity. However, it requires a certain degree of knowledge and experience on the part of the examiner.

Howitt et al. (1967) developed one of the first indices to consider the aesthetic aspects of malocclusion: the *Eastman Esthetic Index* (EEI). In spite of its innovation in measuring the degree of aesthetic impact associated with the malocclusion, it has not achieved such widespread use as other indices.

Salzmann (1967) was one of the first authors to be truly concerned about the patients' own perception of their malocclusion and about the impact and importance of orthodontics, and even of malocclusion, in society. As a result, he published the *Handicapping Malocclusion Assessment Record* (HMAR) index (Salzmann, 1968). The aim was to assess the patients' orthodontic treatment need, classifying the individuals examined according to the level of severity of the problem. This is considered an index with high reproducibility, as it does not use millimetrical measurements but concerns itself with determining functional problems that genuinely constitute an obstacle to the maintenance of oral health and interfere with the patients' proper development owing to their effect on dentofacial aesthetics, mandibular function or speech.

Summers (1971) published the *Occlusal Index* after observing the lack of consensus among orthodontic specialists. This index attempts to classify individuals as objectively as possible and presents clearly epidemiological characteristics. It measures nine occlusal features. Its main distinguishing feature is that it takes the patient's age into account.

Bjork et al. (1964) developed a method with clearly defined variables that can be recorded with good inter-examiner agreement. Based on this method, in 1969 a group of scientists from the World Dental Federation (FDI) Commission on Classification and Statistics of Oral Conditions-Measures of Occlusal Traits (COCSTC-MOT) analyzed the problem of determining occlusal status and developing recording systems for epidemiological purposes. The *Method for Measuring Occlusal Traits* was subsequently developed. This was adopted in 1972 by the FDI (1973) and modified by COCSTC-MOT in collaboration with the WHO, giving rise in 1979 to the final version of the "WHO/FDI Basic Method for Recording of Malocclusion", published in the Bulletin of the WHO (1979). The basic aims of this method, which follows clearly defined criteria, are to determine the prevalence of malocclusion and estimate the treatment needs of the population as a basis for planning orthodontic services.

The *Dental Aesthetic Index* (DAI) created by Cons et al. (1986), is unlike other indices in that the authors based it on the public's perception of dental aesthetics. This index has been used very successfully in numerous studies to assess the prevalence of malocclusion and the orthodontic treatment needs of different population groups. It will be discussed in greater detail in the next section.

The *Index of Orthodontic Treatment Need* (IOTN) described by Brook and Shaw (1989) has achieved widespread recognition both nationally and internationally as an objective method for determining treatment need. This index classifies the patients according to both the degree to which the malocclusion affects their stomatognathic system and their aesthetic perception of their own malocclusion, with the aim of identifying which patients would benefit most from orthodontic treatment (Uçüncü & Ertugay, 2001). A more detailed description is given in section 5.

The *Peer Assessment Rating* (PAR) is a more recent index, developed in Europe in 1992 by Richmond et al. (1992). In their article, the authors explained that it would be very helpful for orthodontists to have an index which would enable them to assess the results on completing the treatment. They considered that the indices developed up to that point lacked sufficient reproducibility and validity. The PAR makes it possible to compare the success of orthodontic treatments and also to predict the severity of cases. To develop this rating, 10 orthodontic specialists assessed 200 models and assigned a value to each of the 11 occlusal features they considered indispensable for evaluating the severity of a malocclusion. The total PAR score is the sum of each of the values of the different occlusal features. The success of a treatment is tested by measuring the PAR index before and after treatment and calculating the difference between the scores. The validity of the study was confirmed by another in which 74 dentists examined 272 dental models and assessed their deviation from the ideal on a scale of 1 to 9. They also calculated the PAR score for each of the models. The correlation between the professionals' opinion and the PAR score was r=0.74, showing that this index is a good predictor of subjective clinical assessment. Subsequently, its validity has also been corroborated by other authors (McGorray et al., 1999).

The latest index reported in the literature is the *Index of Complexity, Outcome and Need* (ICON) developed in 2000 by Daniels and Richmond (2002). Its aim is to bring assessment of need and of the results of orthodontic treatment together in a single index. Its development drew on 97 orthodontists from different countries who gave their subjective opinion of the treatment need, complexity of the treatment and improvement following treatment of 240 initial models and 98 treated models. The criteria employed are the five occlusal features that predicted the expert group's opinion and the IOTN AC (IOTN aesthetic component). Cut-off points were analyzed to determine at what point the index gave an accurate prediction of the specialists' decisions. Good results were obtained for accuracy (85%), sensitivity (85.2%) and specificity (84.4%).

4. Dental Aesthetic Index (DAI)

Cons et al. (1986) described and explained the Dental Aesthetic Index (DAI). The distinctive feature of the DAI is that it is an orthodontic index which relates the clinical and aesthetic components mathematically to produce a single score. It is based on the SASOC (Social Acceptability Scale of Occlusal Conditions) developed earlier by the same authors (Jenny et al., 1980).

The authors wanted to achieve a different index that would be based on the public's perception of dental aesthetics. This was determined through an evaluation of 200 photographs of different occlusal configurations. The 200 cases were chosen, by a random process, from a larger sample of 1337 study models used in a previous study. The 1337 models represented a population of half a million schoolchildren aged between 15 and 18 years from the state of New York. The 200 photographs employed as stimuli for the assessment of dental aesthetics were chosen through a process that ensured that even the most extreme cases were represented. Approximately 2000 adolescents and adults took part in rating the aesthetics of the 200 photographs, each of which showed the models' occlusion in front and side views. The presence and measurement of 49 occlusal features selected by an international committee as being those it was important to consider when developing an orthodontic index were taken into account for each photograph.

Regression analysis was employed to relate the public's assessment of dental aesthetics to the anatomical measurements of the occlusal features that were present in each photograph. This led to the choice of ten occlusal features as the most important ones to take into account in an orthodontic index, insofar as each of them affected the structures of the mouth and influenced dental aesthetics.

This study provided a statistical basis for establishing the value of the regression coefficients used for the ten occlusal features finally chosen for the regression calculations.

All the variables were adjusted in a linear regression model and a predictive equation called the DAI equation was obtained. In the DAI equation, the score for each of the ten DAI components is multiplied by its respective regression coefficient (weighting), the values are added together and a constant, 13, is added to the total. The result of this operation is the DAI score. The DAI equation is as follows:

$\sum$ (DAI Component X Regression Coefficient) + 13

In the DAI equation the regression coefficients are usually rounded off, making it less precise but easier to apply, especially in epidemiological studies. The actual and rounded regression coefficients and constant are shown in Table 1.

The way to measure the ten DAI components correctly is as follows:

1. Number of missing visible teeth (incisors, canines, and premolars in the maxillary and mandibular arches). These are only taken into account if they affect the dental aesthetics, so if the space is closed, if eruption of the permanent tooth is expected or if the missing tooth has been replaced by a dental prosthesis, they should not be counted as missing visible teeth.
2. Assessment of crowding in the incisal segments. The aim is to calculate the existing crowding in the upper anterior and lower anterior sextants. The crowding discrepancy is not measured numerically but only as being present or absent. As a result the score will be 0 if there is no crowding, 1 if there is maxillary or mandibular crowding or 2 if the crowding affects both jaws.
3. Assessment of spacing in the incisal segments. In this case the space between the canines is greater than that required to accommodate the four incisors in a correct alignment. If one or more incisors has a proximal surface without interdental contact, the incisal segment is recorded as spaced. The score will be 0 if there is no spacing, 1 if there is maxillary or mandibular spacing or 2 if the spacing affects both jaws.
4. Measurement of any midline diastema in millimeters. Diastema is a very important occlusal feature from an aesthetic point of view. The midline diastema is defined as the space in millimeters between the two central permanent maxillary incisors when the points of contact are in their normal position.

5. Largest anterior irregularity on the maxilla in millimeters. The largest irregularity, again in millimeters, is measured according to the degree of vestibular-lingual displacement of each tooth in the anterior area of the maxillary arch. As the real crowding discrepancy cannot be measured in terms of millimeters of crowding without taking plaster models, which is not feasible in an epidemiological study, the largest irregularity encountered is recorded.

6. Largest anterior irregularity on the mandible in millimeters. The largest anterior irregularity is measured in millimeters, as for the maxilla.

7. Measurement of anterior maxillary overjet in millimeters. The distance from the labio-incisal edge of the upper incisor to the vestibular surface of the lower incisor. A WHO-type periodontal probe held parallel to the occlusal plane is employed for this measurement.

8. Measurement of anterior mandibular overjet in millimeters. The distance from the incisal edge of the most prominent lower incisor to the labial surface of the corresponding upper incisor.

9. Measurement of vertical anterior openbite. This measures the vertical space between the upper and lower incisors in millimeters.

10. Assessment of anteroposterior molar relation; largest deviation from normal either left or right. The score will be 0 if the occlusal relation is Angle Class I, 1 if the mesial or distal deviation is less than one full cusp and 2 if the mesial or distal deviation is one full cusp or more.

DAI components	Regression Coefficients	
	Actual weights	Rounded weights
1. Number of missing visible teeth (incisors, canines, and premolars in the maxillary and mandibular arches).	5.76	6
2. Assessment of crowding in the incisal segments: 0 = no segments crowded;1 = 1 segment crowded; 2 = 2 segments crowded.	1.15	1
3. Assessment of spacing in the incisal segments: 0 = no segments spaced;1 = 1 segment spaced; 2 = 2 segments spaced.	1.31	1
4. Measurement of any midline diastema in mm.	3.13	3
5. Largest anterior irregularity on the maxilla in mm.	1.34	1
6. Largest anterior irregularity on the mandible in mm.	0.75	1
7. Measurement of anterior maxillary overjet in mm.	1.62	2
8. Measurement of anterior mandibular overjet in mm.	3.68	4
9. Measurement of vertical anterior openbite in mm.	3.69	4
10. Assessment of anteroposterior molar relation; largest deviation from normal either left or right, 0 = normal, 1 = 1/2 cusp either mesial or distal, 2 = 1 full cusp or more either mesial or distal.	2.69	3
CONSTANT	13.36	13

Table 1. Components of the DAI regression equation and their actual and rounded regression coefficients (weights).

Although the DAI was developed for permanent teeth, it can easily be adapted for mixed dentition by simply ignoring missing permanent teeth if these are expected to erupt during the normal time range.

Once the patient's score has been calculated, it can be located on a scale in order to determine its position in relation to the dental aesthetics that are socially most acceptable and least acceptable. The higher the DAI score, the further the occlusal relation is from socially accepted dental aesthetics and the more easily it can be detrimental to the patient.

The DAI has ranges of scores to determine the severity of the malocclusion. A DAI score of 25 or less represents normal occlusion or slight malocclusion. Scores between 26 and 30 indicate moderate malocclusion with questionable treatment need. From 31 to 35, the malocclusion is more serious and treatment is recommended. Scores of 36 or more show severe malocclusion for which treatment is definitely needed.

As mentioned above, although the DAI scale offers these ranges to determine treatment need the scores can be placed on a continuous scale. The continuous scale makes the DAI sufficiently sensitive to differentiate between cases with a greater or lesser need within the same degree of severity. The cutoff points to decide which malocclusions should be treated by the public health services can be modified in view of the available resources.

One of the advantages of the DAI is that it can be obtained in barely 2 minutes, without X-rays, through an oral examination carried out by a trained dental assistant.

DAI components	Component x R. weight	Total
1. Number of missing visible teeth (incisors, canines, and premolars in the maxillary and mandibular arches).	1 missing tooth x 6	6
2. Assessment of crowding in the incisal segments: 0 = no segments crowded;1 = 1 segment crowded; 2 = 2 segments crowded.	1 segment x 1	1
3. Assessment of spacing in the incisal segments: 0 = no segments spaced;1 = 1 segment spaced; 2 = 2 segments spaced.	0 segments x 1	0
4. Measurement of any midline diastema in mm.	0 mm x 3	0
5. Largest anterior irregularity on the maxilla in mm.	3 mm x 1	3
6. Largest anterior irregularity on the mandible in mm.	2 mm x 1	2
7. Measurement of anterior maxillary overjet in mm.	5 mm x 2	10
8. Measurement of anterior mandibular overjet in mm.	0 mm x 4	0
9. Measurement of vertical anterior openbite in mm.	0 mm x 4	0
10. Assessment of anteroposterior molar relation; largest deviation from normal either left or right, 0 = normal, 1 = 1/2 cusp either mesial or distal, 2 = 1 full cusp or more either mesial or distal.	2 (full cusp) x 3	6
Constant		13
DAI score		41

Table 2. This hypothetical case illustrates how the DAI is calculated with the rounded coefficients.

The score for the hypothetical case in Table 2 is 41, which would place the patient in the "orthodontic treatment needed" category.

4.1 Validity and reliability of the DAI

While developing the DAI and after their studies and subsequent publications, Jenny et al. (1993) considered that one of its characteristics was its high degree of validity.

The authors (Jenny & Cons, 1996) tested the reliability of the DAI when measured by trained assistants and found very high intra-class correlation. Although deep overbites that damage the soft tissues are not scored numerically in the DAI, these and other severe congenital conditions are easily recognized by trained personnel, who can refer such cases to orthodontic specialists.

The same authors found that while the acceptability of particular physical features of faces varied widely between different racial and cultural groups, that of dental characteristics remained far more constant among different cultures. This has made it possible to employ the DAI to assess malocclusions in different regions and countries, where it has shown itself to be a quick, simple, reliable index with a high level of validity.

A comparison of an evaluation of 1337 models by orthodontists with the results of the DAI found 88% agreement (Cons et al., 1986). In a prospective study conducted in Australia it was found that a DAI score that indicated treatment need was a good predictor of future orthodontic treatment (Lobb et al., 1994).

One important aspect of the DAI is that it can be measured by trained dental assistants, and this prior screening of the malocclusion severity levels from which patients can be treated reduces the number of first visits by orthodontists employed in public programs.

Numerous studies have suggested that the DAI can be applied universally without any need for modification or adaptation, allowing it to be used independently of the sample in which the study was conducted (Baca-Garcia et al., 2004).

Also, nowadays, the DAI has been included in the latest WHO oral health survey update (1997). The WHO's recommendation of this method for assessing dentofacial anomalies is a major step in its dissemination as a universal method for evaluating malocclusions.

5. IOTN (Index of Orthodontic Treatment Need)

Peter Brook and William Shaw (1989) developed the Orthodontic Treatment Priority (OTP) index, which they later called the IOTN. It was based on a combination of the SCAN or Standardized Continuum of Aesthetic Need (Evans & Shaw, 1987) and the index employed by the Swedish Dental Health Board. The IOTN was subsequently modified by Richmond et al. (1992) and Lunn et al. (1993).

The IOTN consists of two separate components, the aesthetic component (AC) and the dental health component (DHC). It is a method that attempts to determine the degree of malocclusion of a particular patient and that patient's perception of his or her own malocclusion. The novel feature of the IOTN compared to other indices was that it was the first to include a sociopsychological indicator of treatment need.

The two components are analyzed separately and while they cannot be unified to give a single score, they can be combined to classify the patient as needing or not needing orthodontic treatment.

From the start, the authors wanted their index to have two separate components, one to assess the aesthetic impact of the malocclusion and another for the present or potential dental health and functional indications. They also wanted each occlusal feature that contributes to the greater or lesser longevity of the stomatognathic system to be precisely defined, with easily detected and measured levels of severity and cutoff points between them.

Owing to the difficulty in determining the relative contribution of each feature to dental health, the index has to be flexible so that it can be adapted in the light of future research and discoveries.

5.1 The DHC (Dental Health Component) of the IOTN

The DHC (Dental Health Component) is the clinical or dental health component of the IOTN. It is the result of a modification of the index used by the Swedish Dental Health Board (Linder-Aronson, 1974).

The salient feature of this component of the IOTN is that it classifies patients into five distinct grades with clear cutoff points between each, defined according to the occlusal features of each patient and the contribution of each feature to the longevity of the stomatognathic system. In other words, it classifies the occlusal findings that represent the greatest threat to good oral health and function into different grades. Also, it can be obtained directly from examination of the patient or from study models.

One of the main features of this index is that it is not cumulative: it only takes into account the most severe occlusal feature and classifies the patient directly into the appropriate grade. In the same way, it largely ignores the cumulative effect of less severe occlusal features and, consequently, can undervalue certain malocclusions in some individuals.

The DHC has five grades, from Grade 1 (no need for treatment) to Grade 5 (very great need for treatment).

Index of Orthodontic Treatment Need Dental Health Component (IOTN DHC), (Brook & Shaw, 1989).

Grade 5 (Very great)

-   Defects of cleft lip and palate and other craniofacial anomalies.
-   Increased overjet greater than 9 mm.
-   Reverse overjet greater than 3.5 mm with reported masticatory and speech difficulties.
-   Impeded eruption of teeth (with exception of third molars) due to crowding displacement, the presence of supernumerary teeth, retained deciduous teeth, and any pathological cause.
-   Extensive hypodontia with restorative implications (more than one tooth missing in any quadrant) requiring pre-restorative orthodontics.

Grade 4 (Great)

-   Increased overjet greater than 6 mm but less than or equal to 9 mm.

- Reverse overjet greater than 3.5 mm with no reported masticatory or speech difficulties.
- Reverse overjet greater than 1 mm but less than or equal to 3.5 mm with reported masticatory or speech difficulties.
- Anterior or posterior crossbites with greater than 2 mm displacement between retruded contact position and intercuspal position.
- Posterior lingual crossbite with no functional occlusal contact in one or both buccal segments.
- Severe displacement of teeth greater than 4 mm.
- Extreme lateral or anterior open bite greater than 4 mm.
- Increased and complete overbite causing notable indentations on the palate or labial gingivae.
- Less extensive hypodontia requiring prerestorative orthodontics or orthodontic space closure to obviate the need for a prosthesis (not more than 1 tooth missing in any quadrant).

Grade 3 (moderate)

- Increased overjet greater than 3.5 mm but less than or equal to 6 mm with incompetent lips at rest.
- Reverse overjet greater than 1 mm but less than or equal to 3.5 mm.
- Increased and complete overbite with gingival contact but without indentations or signs of trauma.
- Anterior or posterior crossbites with less than or equal to 2 mm but greater than 1 mm discrepancy between retruded contact position and intercuspal position.
- Moderate lateral or anterior open bite greater than 2 mm but less than or equal to 4 mm.
- Moderate displacement of teeth greater than 2 mm but less than or equal to 4 mm.

Grade 2 (little)

- Increased overjet greater than 3.5 mm but less than or equal to 6 mm with lips competent at rest.
- Reverse overjet greater than 0 mm but less than or equal to 1 mm.
- Increased overbite greater than 3.5 mm with no gingival contact.
- Anterior or posterior crossbite with less than or equal to 1 mm displacement between retruded contact position and intercuspal position.
- Small lateral or anterior open bites greater than 1 mm but less than or equal to 2 mm.
- Prenormal or postnormal occlusions with no other anomalies.
- Mild displacement oh teeth greater than 1 mm but less than or equal to 2 mm.

Grade 1 (None)

- Other variations in occlusion including displacement less than or equal to 1 mm.

Lunn et al. (1993) conducted a study to assess the use of the IOTN. They concluded that this index is a very valid tool for public administration purposes but suggested the need for certain modifications to make it quicker and easier to use.

Their suggestions included reducing the number of IOTN DHC grades to three in order to improve its reliability. These proposals were accepted by the Manchester team that had developed the IOTN.

- DHC 1-2   Little or no need for treatment
- DHC 3   Moderate need for treatment
- DHC 4-5   Great need for treatment

These modifications make it much easier to determine the treatment need of a population.

Burden et al. (2001) then proposed a further modification specifically for epidemiological studies, reducing the number of grades to two to make the IOTN DHC easier to use and to increase its validity and reliability.

- DHC 1-2-3   No need for treatment
- DHC 4-5   Need for treatment

They also decided to use the acronym MOCDO (Missing teeth, Overjet, Crossbites, Displacement of contact points, Overbite) to speed up the process and select the patients that need treatment.

This simplifies training and use. According to this modification, those with the following conditions need treatment:

- M (missing teeth): Hypodontia requiring prerestorative orthodontics or space closure. Impeded eruption of teeth. The presence of supernumerary teeth or retained deciduous teeth.
- O (overjet): Overjet greater than 6 millimeters. Reverse overjet greater than 3.5 millimeters without masticatory or speech difficulties. Reverse overjet greater than 1 millimeter but less than or equal to 3.5 millimeters with masticatory or speech difficulties.
- C (crossbites): Anterior or posterior crossbites with more than 2 millimeters displacement between retruded contact position and maximum intercuspal position.
- D (Displacement of contact points): Displacement of contact points greater than 4 millimeters.
- O (Overbite): Lateral or anterior open bite greater than 4 millimeters. Deep overbite causing gingival or palatal traumatic injury.

For the reasons mentioned above this modified IOTN is recommended for epidemiological studies, although it is not useful for administrative purposes because, having only two grades, the patients cannot be classified on a scale of malocclusion severity, so it is more difficult to adjust the resources to the needs.

5.2 The AC (Aesthetic Component) of the IOTN

Since one of the main reasons for undergoing orthodontic treatment is aesthetic, it was considered that the aesthetic component ought to be represented in a diagnostic tool or an index (Alkhatib et al., 2005) and that the patients' perception of their own malocclusion needed to be taken into account.

The aesthetic component (AC) employs the SCAN Index (Evans & Shaw, 1987). It consists of an illustrated scale showing ten grades of dental aesthetics and is employed to determine each patient's aesthetic perception of his or her own malocclusion. To design this index, 1000 intraoral photographs of 12-year-old children were collected and placed in order after a lengthy study (Brook & Shaw, 1989). The photographs were rated by six non-dental judges. The result was a scale of ten black and white photographs showing different levels of dental attractiveness, ranging from photograph 1, the most aesthetic, to number 10, the least aesthetic (Uçüncü & Ertugay, 2001).

The patient has to look at his or her mouth in a mirror and identify it with one of the ten photographs in the scale. In this way, each patient's perception of his or her malocclusion can be observed.

To make the IOTN quicker and easier to use and improve its reliability, Lunn et al. (1993) proposed reducing the number of IOTN AC grades from 10 to 3. These proposals were accepted by the Manchester team that had developed the IOTN.

- AC 1-4   Little or no need for treatment
- AC 5-7   Moderate need for treatment
- AC 8-10   Great need for treatment

Nowadays, for practical and epidemiological purposes only two grades are considered: patients who identify with photographs 1 to 7 do not need treatment, while those who identify with photographs 8 to 10 do need treatment. It should be pointed out that in most cases, almost no patients identify their own teeth with the great orthodontic treatment need group (photographs 8-10). It is also considered to be no easy task for patients to decide which of the 10 photographs most resemble their own teeth, especially when they are very young.

In practice, the two components of the IOTN are determined separately and an individual is considered to need treatment if the IOTN DHC grade is 4 or 5 or the IOTN AC is in the grades 8-10 group. In either of these two situations the child needs orthodontic treatment for either dental health reasons (DHC) or for exclusively aesthetic reasons (AC). However, according to the modified IOTN developed by Burden et al. (2001), when this is employed in epidemiological studies both components are required, in other words, DHC grades 4-5 and AC grades 8-10.

5.3 Validity and reliability of the IOTN

When designing and testing the IOTN, Brook and Shaw (1989) observed that the reproducibility of this index was particularly good when measured under suitable conditions, and slightly less good when measured, for example, in schools.

Richmond et al. (1995) confirmed the validity and reliability of the IOTN in a study in which 74 dentists and orthodontists assessed the treatment need of a total of 256 models of orthodontic patients representing all types of malocclusion. The Spearman coefficient for the aesthetic component was 0.84 and that of the dental health component was 0.64.

Brook and Shaw claim good intra- and inter-examiner reproducibility when the IOTN AC is assessed by a dentist. However, according to Holmes (1992), the patients' perception tends to be more optimistic than that of the professionals. Nevertheless, the use of the IOTN AC has been the subject of some controversy in recent years. This is because of the lack of correlation between the dental health component (DHC) and the aesthetic component (AC), as found by Soh and Sandham (2004) in a study of an adult Asian population and by Hassan (2006) in a region of Saudi Arabia. Also, some authors such as Svedström-Oristo et al. (2009) have described certain problems when asking patients, both children and young adults, to identify their mouths with one of the 10 photographs employed as stimuli.

According to Alkhatib et al. (2005), the IOTN is not only valid and reliable but is also sensitive to the needs of patients and accepted both by the patients themselves and by the professionals who employ it. Hamdam (2004) confirmed the validity and reliability of the IOTN. Mandall et al. (2000) and Birkeland et al. (1996) concluded that it is a reproducible and reliable index.

A recent study by Johansson and Follin (2009) showed that the clinical criterion employed by 272 Swedish orthodontists was in good agreement with the results of the IOTN DHC. The main differences were found in IOTN grade 3, as the orthodontists considered most of the malocclusions in this grade to be in need of treatment.

However, O'Brien et al. (1993) found large differences in the choice of the different grades of need in both the DHC and the AC. Turbill et al. (1996) concluded that the IOTN is essentially an epidemiological index that has limitations when assessing the treatment needs of individual patients.

The IOTN is currently employed in the United Kingdom for prioritizing public orthodontic care services. Its reliability and validity have been extensively proved, it is simple and easy to use, and it is also one of the most-often cited indices in the literature.

6. The epidemiology of treatment need

Appropriate assessment and measurement of malocclusions is essential in epidemiological studies in order to ascertain the prevalence and incidence of occlusal alterations among the population. There are certainly many indices and measures for assessing malocclusion, but the DAI and the IOTN are the best known and most widely used owing to their manageability and proven validity.

Tables 3 and 4 show a number of malocclusion prevalence studies conducted since the year of publication of each of these indices up to the present.

On examining the main studies it will be seen that both the DAI and the IOTN have been used to a greater extent in cross-sectional studies with large samples, generally randomly selected, although it will be observed that they meet the requirements for epidemiological or prevalence studies. While the IOTN is used to a greater extent in Europe, The DAI is employed to a similar extent throughout the world, though least in Europe. However, whereas the IOTN is employed more in child/adolescent populations, the DAI is more often employed in adolescent/adult ones.

As noted above, comparison between the different studies is very complicated. The first reason is that they employ different methods and their data collection criteria are sometimes not sufficiently well explained. Examination of the studies shows that they use different indices, so although they measure the same condition (malocclusion prevalence or treatment need), they do not measure it in the same way or consider the same occlusal features. Obviously, also, the different studies were conducted in different populations, with differing sample sizes, ages and geographical origins. For all these reasons, it is possible to make comparisons but prudence is required when drawing conclusions. Epidemiological studies of malocclusion prevalence and orthodontic treatment need in large, representative samples continue to be necessary in order to effect more rigorous comparisons.

Authors (publication year)	Country	n	Age	DHC(4-5)	AC(8-10)
Brook and Shaw (1989)	United Kingdom	222	11-12	32.7%	5.4%
So and Tang (1993)	Hong Kong	100	19-20	53%	-
So and Tang (1993)	China	100	20	52%	-
Burden and Holmes (1994)	United Kingdom	874 955	11-12	31% 32%	12% 8.5%
Tuominen et al. (1995)	Finland	89	16-19	11.2%	-
Tang and So (1995)	Hong Kong	105	18-22	54.2%	-
Birkeland et al. (1996)	Norway	359	11	26.1%	9%
Otuyemi et al. (1997)	Nigeria	704	12-18	12.6%	-
Riedmann and Berg (1999)	Germany	88	20	60.2%	60%
Tickle et al. (1999)	United Kingdom	7888	14	26.2%	-
Cooper et al. (2000)	United Kingdom	142	19	21%	12.8%
Kerosuo et al. (2000)	Finland	281	18-19	15%	0%
Cooper et al. (2000)	United Kingdom	314	11	34%	4%
Johnson et al. (2000)	New Zealand	294	10	31.3%	3.8%
Mandall et al. (2000)	United Kingdom	434	14-15	18%	6%
Uçüncü y Ertugay (2001)	Turkey	250	11-14	38.8%	4.8%
Abdullah and Rock (2001)	Malaysia	5112	12-13	30%	-
Hamdam (2001)	Jordan	320	14-17	28	-
Hunt et al. (2002)	United Kingdom	215	17-43	-	2.8%
De Olivera and Sheiham (2003)	Brazil	1675	15-16	22%	-
Klages et al. (2004)	Germany	148	18-30	-	0%
Flores-Mir et al. (2004)	Canada	329	18-20	-	2%
Soh and Sandham (2004)	Singapore	339	17-22	50.1 %	29.2%
Kerosuo et al. (2004)	Kuwait	139	14-18	28.1%	1.4%
Abu Alhaija et al. (2004)	Jordan	1002	12-14	34%	-
Tausche et al. (2004)	Germany	1975	6-8	26.2%	21.5%
Mugonzibwa et al. (2004)	Tanzania	386	9-18	22%	11%
Hamdam (2004)	Jordan	103	15	71%	16.7%
Kerosuo et al. (2004)	Kuwait	139	14-18	28%	2%
Hlonga et al. (2004)	Tanzania	643	15-16	3-13%	-
Soh et al. (2005)	Singapore	339	17-22	50.1%	29.2%
Alkhatib et al. (2005)	United Kingdom	3500	12-14	15%	2.1%
Mandall et al. (2005)	United Kingdom	525	11-12	44.8%	2.7%
Klages et al. (2006)	Germany	194	18-30	-	8.8%

Authors (publication year)	Country	n	Age	DHC(4-5)	AC(8-10)
Bernabé and Flores-Mir (2006b)	Peru	281	16-25	29.9%	1.8%
Hassan (2006)	Saudi Arabia	743	17-24	71.6%	16.1%
Souames et al. (2006)	France	511	9-12	21.3%	7%
Chestnutt et al. (2006)	United Kingdom	2595 / 2142	12 / 15	35% / 21%	- / -
Nobile et al. (2007)	Italy	1000	11-15	59.5%	3.2%
Ngom et al. (2007)	Senegal	665	12-13	42.6%	3.3%
Manzanera et al. (2009)	Spain	665	12 / 15-16	21.8% / 17.1%	4.4% / 2.4%
Svedström-Oristo et al. (2009)	Finland	434	16-25	-	2%
Puertes-Fernández et al. (2010)	Algeria	248	12	18.1%	13.7%
Hassan and Amin (2010)	Saudi Arabia	366	21-25	29.2%	-

Table 3. Studies of different populations using the IOTN (DHC/AC)

Authors (publication year)	Country	n	Age	Treatment Need (≥31)
Estioko et al. (1994)	Australia	268	12-16	24.1%
Katoh et al. (1998)	Japan / Taiwan	1029 / 176	15-29 / 18-24	30.1% / 25.9%
Otuyemi et al. (1999)	Nigeria	703	12-18	9.2%
Johnson et al. (2000)	New Zealand	294	10	55.4%
Chi et al. (2000)	New Zealand	150	10	47%
Abdullah and Rock (2001)	Malaysia	5112	12-13	24.1%
Esa et al. (2001)	Malaysia	1519	12-13	24.1%
Onyeaso et al. (2003)	Nigeria	64	16-45	48.4%
Baca-García et al. (2004)	Spain	744	14-20	21.1%
Onyeaso (2004)	Nigeria	136	6-18	50%
Onyeaso (2005)	Nigeria	577	12-17	22.7%
van Wyk and Drummond (2005)	South Africa	6142	12	31%
Frazão and Narvai (2006)	Brazil	13801	12-18	18%
Bernabé and Flores-Mir (2006a)	Peru	267	16-25	32.6%
Marques et al. (2007)	Brazil	600	13-15	53.3%
Hamamci et al. (2009)	Turkey	841	17-26	21.5%
Manzanera et al. (2010)	Spain	655	12 / 15-16	21.2% / 16.1%
Puertes-Fernández et al. (2010)	Algeria	248	12	13.2%

Table 4. Studies of different populations using the DAI

7. Conclusions

Many very different indices have been developed for classifying malocclusions according to their severity or level of treatment need. Although a certain consensus has been reached on the features that the ideal index should possess, controversy continues over which should be used for this purpose.

Evidently, patients often seek orthodontic treatment but present considerable variations in malocclusion. The wide range of situations between ideal occlusion and very severe malocclusion make it very difficult to establish the precise limits of what should and should not be considered treatment need. Consequently, ascertaining the real malocclusion prevalence and establishing reliable comparisons concerning their frequency in different populations is by no means simple. Also, as there is also no unanimous criterion for deciding what to consider malocclusion, its real frequency cannot be established.

In this chapter we have presented a large number of orthodontic treatment need indices. However, the two indices that are currently most often used for epidemiological studies are the DAI and the IOTN. Hlonga et al. (2004) and Liu et al. (2011) have observed a significant correlation between the two indices. Nevertheless, high correlation does not necessarily imply high agreement (Manzanera et al., 2010). In epidemiological studies this is not a particularly important problem because both are valid methods for determining the orthodontic treatment need of a population, but when they are applied in individual cases, the choice of DAI or IOTN will lead to the appearance of both false negatives and false positives.

Comparison of these two indices finds similarities and differences. Both comprise two components, one anatomical and the other aesthetic, both measure occlusion features proposed by experts and both attempt to identify the individuals with the greatest treatment need in public programs. Although most of the features they measure are identical, each feature is rated differently in the two indices. The advantage of the DAI is that the aesthetic perception is linked to the anatomical assessment through regression analysis to produce a single score, whereas the IOTN has two components that cannot be unified. Also, the DAI offers a continuous scoring system, so it can classify different degrees of malocclusion within each of the pre-established levels. The IOTN cannot establish a continuous order within each grade, so it is more complicated to use for public health programs. In the DAI, unlike the IOTN, the occlusal features examined are different according to whether it is the primary dentition, mixed dentition or permanent dentition that is being measured, and since its design is more suitable for permanent teeth, it leads to the use of more than one epidemiological index.

It would appear, agreeing with some other authors, that DAI is more useful for administrative purposes, in other words, when the budget is limited and the patients must be placed in strict order of severity in order to give priority to those in most need of treatment. This is possible because the DAI scale is continuous, whereas the IOTN makes not distinctions within grades. The IOTN, however, being easily and quickly obtained, is more effective in epidemiological studies, to determine the percentage of the population in need of treatment without establishing priorities.

The great value that society sets on aesthetics nowadays, the importance that patients themselves ascribe to their malocclusions and the extent to which their condition affects their quality of life must not be forgotten. In recent years particular attention has been paid to surveys that attempt to measure the way in which malocclusion affects a person's quality of life; these include studies by De Baets et al. (2011), Liu et al. (2011) and Agou et al. (2011). Such surveys should be employed in decision-making as complementary tools to the different orthodontic treatment need indices.

8. References

Abdullah, M.S. & Rock, W.P. (2001), Assessment of orthodontic treatment need in 5,112 Malaysian children using the IOTN and DAI indices. *Community Dent Health*, Vol.18, No.4, pp. 242-248.

Abu Alhaija, E.S.; Al-Nimri, K.S. & Al-Khateeb, S.N. (2004). Orthodontic treatment need and demand in 12-14-year-old north Jordanian school children. *Eur J Orthod*, Vol.26, No.3, pp. 261-263.

Ackerman, J.L. & Proffit, W.R. (1969). Characteristics of malocclusion: a modern approach to classification and diagnosis. *Am J Orthod*, Vol.56, No.5, pp. 443-454.

Agou, S.; Locker, D.; Muirhead, V.; Tompson, B. & Streiner, D.L. (2011). Does psychological well-being influence oral-health-related quality of life reports in children receiving orthodontic treatment?. *Am J Orthod Dentofacial Orthop*, Vol.139, No.3, pp. 369-377.

Alkhatib, M.N.; Bedi, R.; Foster, C.; Jopanputra, P. & Allan, S. (2005). Ethnic variations in orthodontic treatment need in London schoolchildren. *BMC Oral Health*, 27;5:8.

Angle, E.H. (1899). Classification of malocclusion. *Dent Cosmos*, Vol.41, pp. 248-264.

Andrews, L.F. (1972). The six keys to normal occlusion. *Am J Orthod*, Vol.62, pp.296-309.

Baca-Garcia, A.; Bravo, M.; Baca, P.; Baca, A. & Junco, P. (2004). Malocclusions and orthodontic treatment needs in a group of Spanish adolescents using the Dental Aesthetic Index. *Int Dent J*, Vol.54, no.3, pp. 138-142.

Bernabé, E.; Flores-Mir, C. (2006a). Orthodontic treatment need in Peruvian young adults evaluated through dental aesthetic index. *Angle Orthod*, Vol.76, No.3, pp. 417-421.

Bernabé, E. & Flores-Mir, C. (2006b). Normative and self-perceived orthodontic treatment need of a Peruvian university population. *Head Face Med*, 3;2:22.

Birkeland, K.; Boe, O.E. & Wisth, P.J. (1996). Orthodontic concern among 11-year-old children and their parents compared with orthodontic treatment need assessed by index of orthodontic treatment need. *Am J Orthod Dentofacial Orthop*, Vol.110, No.2, pp. 197-205.

Björk, A.; Krebs A.A. & Solow, B. (1964). A method for epidemiological registration of malocclusion. *Acta Odontol Scand*, Vol.35, pp. 161-165.

Bravo, L.A. (2003). Naturaleza de la maloclusión y justificación del tratamiento ortodóncico, In: Manual de Ortodoncia, Bravo, L.A., pp. (25-52), Editorial Síntesis, Madrid.

Brook, P.H. & Shaw, W.C. (1989). The development of an index of orthodontic treatment priority. Europ J Orthod, Vol.11, pp. 309-320.

Burden, D.J. & Holmes, A. (1994). The need for orthodontic treatment in the child population of the United Kingdom. *Eur J Orthod*, Vol.16, No.5, pp.395-399.

Burden, D.J.; Pine, C.M. & Burnside, G. (2001). Modified IOTN: an orthodontic treatment need index for use in oral health surveys. *Community Dent Oral Epidemiol*, Vol.29, pp. 220-225.

Canut, J.A. (2 Ed.). (1988). Concepto de ortodoncia, In: *Ortodoncia clínica y terapéutica*, Canut, J.A., pp. (1-16), Masson, Barcelona.

Chestnutt, I.G.; Burden, D.J.; Steele, J.G.; Pitts, N.B.; Nuttall, N.M. & Morris, A.J. (2006). The orthodontic condition of children in the United Kingdom, 2003. *Br Dent J*, Vol.200, No.11, pp. 609-612.

Chi, J.; Johnson, M. & Harkness, M. (2000). Age changes in orthodontic treatment need: a longitudinal study of 10- and 13-year-old children, using the Dental Aesthetic Index. *Aust Orthod J*, Vol.16, No.3, pp. 150-156.

Cons, N.C.; Jenny, J. & Kohout, F.J. (1986). DAI: The Dental Aesthetic Index. Iowa City, Iowa: College of Dentistry, University of Iowa.

Cooper, S.; Mandall, N.A.; DiBiase, D. & Shaw, W.C. (2000). The reliability of the Index of Orthodontic Treatment Need over time. *J Orthod*, Vol.27, No.1, pp. 47-53.

Daniels, C. & Richmond, S. (2000). The development of the index of complexity, outcome and need (ICON). *J Orthod*, Vol. 27, No.2, pp. 149-162.

De Oliveira, C.M. & Sheiham, A. (2003). The relationship between normative orthodontic treatment need and oral health-related quality of life. *Community Dent Oral Epidemiol*, Vol.31, No.6, pp. 426-436.

De Baets, E.; Lambrechts, H.; Lemiere, J.; Diya, L. & Willems, G. (2011). Impact of self-esteem on the relationship between orthodontic treatment need and oral health-related quality of life in 11- to 16-year-old children. *Eur J Orthod*, [Epub ahead of print].

Draker, H.L. (1960). Handicapping labio-lingual deviation: A proposed index for public health purposes. *Am J Orthod*, Vol.46, pp. 295-305.

Dewey, M. & Anderson G.M. (6 Ed.). (1942). *Practical Orthodontics*, C.V. Mosby Company, St. Louis, Missouri.

Esa, R.; Razak, I.A. & Allister, J.H. (2001). Epidemiology of malocclusion and orthodontic treatment need of 12-13-year-old Malaysian schoolchildren. *Community Dent Health*, Vol.18, No.1, pp. 31-36.

Estioko, L.J.; Wright, F.A. & Morgan, M.V. (1994). Orthodontic treatment need of secondary schoolchildren in Heidelberg, Victoria: an epidemiologic study using the Dental Aesthetic Index. *Community Dent Health*, Vol.11, No.3, pp. 147-151.

Evans, M.R. & Shaw, W.C. (1987). Preliminary evaluation of an illustrated scale for rating dental attractiveness. *Eur J Orthod*, Vol.9, pp. 314-318.

Federation Dentaire Internationale (1973). A method for measuring occlusal traits, commission on classification and statistics for oral conditions. Working Group 2 on dentofacial anomalies, 1969-1972. *Int Dent J*, Vol.23, pp. 530-537.

Flores-Mir, C.; Major, P.W. & Salazar, F.R. (2004). Self-perceived orthodontic treatment need evaluated through 3 scales in a university population. *J Orthod*; Vol.31, No.4, pp. 329-334.

Frazão, P. & Narvai, P.C. (2006). Socio-environmental factors associated with dental occlusion in adolescents. *Am J Orthod Dentofacial Orthop*, Vol.129, No.6, pp. 809-816.

Grainger, R.M. (1967). Orthodontic Treatment priority index. *Vital Health Stat*; Vol.2, pp. 1-49.

Hamamci, N.; Başaran, G. & Uysal, E. (2009). Dental Aesthetic Index scores and perception of personal dental appearance among Turkish university students. *Eur J Orthod*, Vol.31, No.2, pp. 168-173.

Hamdan, A.M. (2001). Orthodontic treatment need in Jordanian school children. *Community Dent Health*, Vol.18, No.3, pp. 177-180.

Hamdan, A.M. (2004). The relationship between patient, parent and clinician perceived need and normative orthodontic treatment need. *Eur J Orthod*, Vol.26, No.3, pp. 265-271.

Hassan, A.H. (2006). Orthodontic treatment needs in the western region of Saudi Arabia: a research report. *Head Face Med*, 18;2:2.

Hassan, A.H. & Amin, Hel-S. (2010). Association of orthodontic treatment needs and oral health-related quality of life in young adults. *Am J Orthod Dentofacial Orthop*, Vol.137, No.1, pp. 42-47.

Hlongwa, P.; Beane, R.A.; Seedat, A.K. & Owen, C.P. (2004). Orthodontic treatment needs: comparison of two indices. *SADJ*, Vol.59, No.10, pp. 421-424.

Howitt, J.W.; Stricker, G. & Henderson, R. (1967). Eastman Esthetic Index. *N Y State Dent J*, Vol.33, No.4, pp. 215-220.

Hunt, O.; Hepper, P.; Johnston, C.; Stevenson, M. & Burden, D. (2002). The Aesthetic Component of the Index of Orthodontic Treatment Need validated against lay opinion. *Eur J Orthod*, Vol.24, No.1, pp. 53-59.

Jenny, J.; Cons, N.C.; Kohout, F.J. & Frazier, P.J. (1980). Test of a method to determine socially acceptable occlusal conditions. *Community Dent Oral Epidemiol*, Vol.8, No.8, pp. 424-433.

Jenny, J.; Cons, N.C.; Kohout, F.J. & Jakobsen, J. (1993). Predicting handicapping malocclusion using the Dental Aesthetic Index (DAI). *Int Dent J*, Vol.43, pp. 128-132.

Jenny, J. & Cons, N.C. (1996). Establishing malocclusion severity levels on the Dental Aesthetic Index (DAI) scale. *Australian Dent J*, Vol.41, pp. 43-46.

Johansson, A.M. & Follin, M.E. (2009). Evaluation of the Dental Health Component, of the Index of Orthodontic Treatment Need, by Swedish orthodontists. *Eur J Orthod*, Vol.31, No.2, pp. 184-188.

Johnson, M.; Harkness, M.; Crowther, P. & Herbison, P. (2000). A comparison of two methods of assessing orthodontic treatment need in the mixed dentition: DAI and IOTN. *Aust Orthod J*, Vol.16, No.2, pp. 82-87.

Katoh, Y.; Ansai, T. & Takehar, T. (1998). A comparison of DAI scores and characteristics of occlusal traits in three ethnic groups of Asian origin. *Int Dent J*, Vol.48, pp. 405-411.

Kerosuo, H.; Kerosuo, E., Niemi, M. & Simola, H. (2000). The need for treatment and satisfaction with dental appearance among young Finnish adults with and without a history of orthodontic treatment. *J Orofac Orthop*, Vol.61, No.5, pp. 330-340.

Kerosuo, H.; Al Enezi, S.; Kerosuo, E. & Abdulkarim, E. (2004). Association between normative and self-perceived orthodontic treat- ment need among Arab high school students. *Am J Orthod Dentofacial Orthop*, Vol.125, pp. 373-378.

Klages, U.; Bruckner, A. & Zentner, A. (2004). Dental aesthetics, self-awareness, and oral health-related quality of life in young adults. *Eur J Orthod*, Vol.26, No.5, pp. 507-514.

Klages, U.; Claus, N.; Wehrbein, H. & Zentner, A. (2006). Development of a questionnaire for assessment of the psychosocial impact of dental aesthetics in young adults. *Eur J Orthod*, Vol.28, No.2, pp. 103-111.

Kiekens, R.M.; Maltha, J.C.; van't Hof, M.A. & Kuijpers-Jagtman, A.M. (2006). Objective measures as indicators for facial esthetics in white adolescents. *Angle Orthod*, Vol.76, No.4, pp. 551-556.

Kok, Y.V.; Mageson, P.; Harradine, N.W. & Sprod, A.J. (2004). Comparing a quality of life measure and the Aesthetic Component of the Index of Orthodontic Treatment Need (IOTN) in assessing orthodontic treatment need and concern. *J Orthod*, Vol.31, No.4, pp. 312-318.

Lewis, E.A.; Albino, J.E.; Cunat, J.J. & Tudesco, L.A. (1982). Reliability and validity of clinical assessments of malocclusion. *Am J Orthod*, Vol.81, pp. 473-477.

Linder-Aronson, S. (1974). Orthodontics in the Swedish Public Dental Health System. Transactions of the European Orthodontic Society 233-240.

Liu, Z.; McGrath, C. & Hagg, U. (2011). Associations between orthodontic treatment need and oral health-related quality of life hmong young adults: does it dependo on how toy assess them? *Community Dent Oral Epidemiol*, Vol.39, pp. 137-144.

Lischer, B.E. (1912). Principles and methods of orthodontics. Lea & Febiger. Filadelfia, Pensilvannia.

Lobb, W.K.; Ismail, A.I.; Andrews, C.L. & Spracklin, T.E. (1994). Evaluation of orthodontic treatment using Dental Aesthetic Index. *Am J Othod Dentofac Othop*, Vol.106, No.1, pp. 70-75.

Lunn, H.; Richmond, S. & Mitropoulos, C. (1993). The use of the index of Orthodontic Treatment Need (IOTN) as a public health tool: a pilot study. *Community Dent Health*, Vol.10, pp. 111-121.

Mandall, N.A.; McCord, J.F.; Blinkhorn, A.S.; Worthington, H.V. & O'Brien, K.D. (2000). Perceived aesthetic impact of malocclusion and oral self-perceptions in 14-15-year-old Asian and Caucasian children in greater Manchester. *Eur J Orthod*, Vol.22, No.2, pp. 175-183.

Mandall, N.A.; Wright, J.; Conboy, F.; Kay, E., Harvey, L. & O'Brien, K.D. (2005). Index of orthodontic treatment need as a predictor of orthodontic treatment uptake. *Am J Orthod Dentofacial Orthop*, Vol.128, No.6, pp. 703-707.

Manzanera, D.; Montiel-Company, J.M.; Almerich-Silla, J.M. & Gandía, J.L. (2009). Orthodontic treatment need in Spanish schoolchildren: an epidemiological study using the Index of Orthodontic Treatment Need. *Eur J Orthod*, Vol.31, No.2, pp. 180-183.

Manzanera, D.; Montiel-Company, J.M.; Almerich-Silla, J.M. & Gandía, J.L. (2010). Diagnostic agreement in the assessment of orthodontic treatment need using the Dental Aesthetic Index and the Index of Orthodontic Treatment Need. *Eur J Orthod*, Vol.32, No.2, pp.193-198.

Marques, C.R.; Couto, G.B.; Orestes Cardoso, S. (2007). Assessment of orthodontic treatment need in Brazilian schoolchildren according to the Dental Aesthetic Index (DAI). *Community Dent Health*, Vol.24, No.3, pp. 145-148.

McGorray, S.P.; Wheeler, T.T.; Keeling, S.D.; Yurkiewicz, L.; Taylor, M.G. & King, G.J. (1999). Evaluation of orthodontists' perception of treatment need and the peer assessment rating (PAR) index. *The Angle Orthodontist*, Vol.69, No.4, pp. 325-333.

Mugonzibwa, E.A.; Kuijpers-Jagtman, A.M.; Van 't Hof, M.A. & Kikwilu, E.N. (2004). Perceptions of dental attractiveness and orthodontic treatment need among Tanzanian children. *Am J Orthod Dentofacial Orthop*, Vol. 125, No.4, pp. 426-433.

Nobile, C.G., Pavia, M.; Fortunato, L. & Angelillo, I.F. (2007). Prevalence and factors related to malocclusion and orthodontic treatment need in children and adolescents in Italy. *Eur J Public Health*, Vol.17, No.6, pp. 637-641.

Ngom, P.I.; Diagne, F.; Dieye, F.; Diop-Ba, K. & Thiam, F. (2007). Orthodontic treatment need and demand in Senegalese school children aged 12-13 years. An appraisal using IOTN and ICON. *Angle Orthod*, Vol.77, No.2, pp. 323-330.

O'Brien, K.D.; Shaw, W.C. & Roberts, C.T. (1993). The use of occlusal indices in assessing the provision of orthodontic treatment by the hospital orthodontic service of England and Wales. *Br J Orthod*, Vol.20, pp.25-35.

Onyeaso, C.O.; Arowojolu, M.O. & Taiwo, J.O. (2003). Periodontal status of orthodontic patients and the relationship between dental aesthetic index and community periodontal index of treatment need. *Am J Orthod Dentofacial Orthop*, Vol.124, No.6, pp. 714-720.

Onyeaso, C.O. (2004). Orthodontic treatment need of Nigerian outpatients assessed with the Dental Aesthetic Index. *Aust Orthod J*, Vol.20, No.1, pp. 19-23.

Onyeaso, C.O. & Sanu, O.O. (2005). Perception of personal dental appearance in Nigerian adolescents. *Am J Orthod Dentofacial Orthop*, Vol.127, No.6, pp. 700-706.

Otuyemi, O.D.; Ugboko, V.I.; Adekoya-Sofowora, C.A. & Ndukwe, K.C. (1997). Unmet orthodontic treatment need in rural Nigerian adolescents. *Community Dent Oral Epidemiol*, Vol.25, No.5, pp. 363-366.

Otuyemi, O.D.; Ogunyinka, A.; Dosumu, O.; Cons, N.C. & Jenny, J. (1999). Malocclusion and orthodontic treatment need of secondary school students in Nigeria according to the dental aesthetic index (DAI). *Int Dent J*; Vol.49, No.4, pp. 203-210.

Parker, W.S. (1998). The HLD index and the index question. *Am J Orthod Dentofacial Orthop*; Vol.114, pp. 134-141.

Prahl-Andersen, B. (1978). The need for orthodontic treatment. *Angle Orthod*; Vol.48, No1. pp. 1-9.

Puertes-Fernández, N.; Montiel-Company, J.M.; Almerich-Silla, J.M. & Manzanera, D. (2010). Orthodontic treatment need in a 12-year-old population in the Western Sahara. *Eur J Orthod*, [Epub ahead of print].

Richmond, S.; Shaw, W.C.; O'Brien, K.D.; Buchanan, I.B.; Jones, R.; Stephens, C.D.; Roberts, C.T. & Andrews, M. (1992). The development of the PAR Index (Peer Assessment Rating): reliability and validity. *Europ J Orthod*, Vol.14, No.2, pp. 125-139.

Richmond, S.; Shaw, W.C.; O'Brien, K.D.; Buchanan, I.B.; Stephens, C.D.; Andrews, M. & Roberts, C.T. (1995). The relationship between the index of orthodontic treatment need and consensus opinion of a panel of 74 dentists. *Br Dent J*, Vol.178, pp. 370-374.

Richmond, S.; Daniels, C.P.; Fox, N. & Wright, J. (1997). The professional perception of orthodontic treatment complexity. *Br Dent J*, Vol.183, No.10, pp. 371-375.

Riedmann, T. & Berg, R. (1999). Retrospective evaluation of the outcome of orthodontic treatment in adults. *J Orofac Orthop*, Vol.60, No.2, pp. 108-123.

Souames, M.; Bassigny, F.; Zenati, N.; Riordan, P.J. & Boy-Lefevre, M.L. (2006). Orthodontic treatment need in French schoolchildren: an epidemiological study using the Index of Orthodontic Treatment Need. *Eur J Orthod*, Vol.28, No.6, pp. 605-609.

Summers, C.J. (1971). The occlusal index: a system for identifying and scoring occlusal disorders. *Am J Orthod*, Vol.59, No.6, pp. 552-567.

Salzmann, J.A. (1967). Orthodontics and society. *Am J Orthod*; Vol.53, No.10, pp. 783-785.

Shaw, W.C.; Richmond, S. & O'Brien, K.D. (1995). The use of occlusal indices: A European perspective. *Am J Orthod Dentofac Orthop*, Vol.107, pp. 1-10.

Simon, P. (1922). Grundzuge einer systematischen diagnostik der gebiss-anomalien. Meusser. Berlín.

So, L.L. & Tang, E.L. (1993). A comparative study using the Occlusal Index and the Index of Orthodontic Treatment Need. *Angle Orthod*, Vol 63, No.1, pp. 57-64.

Soh, J. & Sandham, A. (2004). Orthodontic treatment need in Asian adult males. *Angle Orthod*, Vol.74, No.6, pp. 769-773.

Soh, J.; Sandham, A. & Chan, Y.H. (2005). Malocclusion severity in Asian men in relation to malocclusion type and orthodontic treatment need. *Am J Orthod Dentofacial Orthop*; Vol.128, No.5, pp. 648-652.

Svedström-Oristo, A.L.; Pietilä, T.; Pietilä, I.; Vahlberg, T.; Alanen, P. & Varrela, J. (2009). Acceptability of dental appearance in a group of Finnish 16- to 25-year-olds. *Angle Orthod*, Vol.79, No.3, pp. 479-483.

Tang, E.L.K. & Wei, S.N.Y. (1993). Recording and measuring malocclusion: a review of the literature. *Am J Orthod Dentofac Orthop*, Vol.103, pp. 344-351.

Tang, E.L. & So, L.L. (1995). Correlation of orthodontic treatment demand with treatment need assessed using two indices. *Angle Orthod*, Vol.65, No.6, pp. 443-450.

Tausche, E., Luck, O. & Harzer, W. (2004). Prevalence of malocclusions in the early mixed dentition and orthodontic treatment need. *Eur J Orthod*, Vol.26, No.3, pp. 237-244.

Tickle, M.; Kay, E.J. & Bearn, D. (1999). Socio-economic status and orthodontic treatment need. *Community Dent Oral Epidemiol*, Vol.27, No.6, pp. 413-418.

Tuominen, M.L.; Nystrom, M. & Tuominen, R.J. (1995). Subjective and objective orthodontic treatment need among orthodontically treated and untreated Finnsih adolescents. *Community Dent Oral Epidemiol*, Vol.23, pp. 286-290.

Turbill, E.A.; Richmond, S. & Wright, J.L. (1996). Assessment of General Dental Services orthodontic standards: the Dental Practice Board's gradings compared to PAR and IOTN. *Br J Orthod*, Vol.23, pp. 211-220.

Uçüncü, N. & Ertugay, E. (2001). The use of the Index of Orthodontic Treatment need (IOTN) in a school population and referred population. *J Orthod*, Vol.28, No.1, pp. 45-52.

Van Kirk, L.E. (1959). Assessment of malocclusion in population groups. *Am J Public Health Nations Health*, Vol.49, pp. 1157-1163.

Van Wyk, P.J. & Drummond, R.J. (2005). Orthodontic status and treatment need of 12-year-old children in South Africa using the Dental Aesthetic Index. *SADJ*; Vol.60, No.8, pp. 334-336.

WHO (1979). Basic method for recording occlusal traits. WHO Bull;57(6):955-61.

WHO (1997). Health Surveys. Basic Methods. Ed. 3 Geneve: World Health Organization.

Are the Orthodontic Basis Wrong? Revisiting Two of the Keys to Normal Oclusion (Crown Inclination and Crown Angulation) in the Andrews Series

C. Jiménez-Caro[1,2], F. de Carlos[1,2], A.A. Suárez[1,3], J.A. Vega[4] and J. Cobo[1,2]

[1]*Instituto Asturiano de Odontología, Oviedo*
[2]*Departamento de Cirugía y Especialidades*
Médico-Quirúrgicas (sección de Odontología), Universidad de Oviedo
[3]*Departamento de Construcción e Ingeniería de la*
Fabricación (Sección de Ingeniería Mecánica), Universidad de Oviedo
[4]*Departamento de Morfología y Biología Celular, Universidad de Oviedo*
Spain

1. Introduction

In the second half of the last century, Lawrence F. Andrews studied a series of 120 casts, of non-orthodontic subjects with ideal patterns of dental occlusion, and established *"The six keys to normal occlusion"*. These were the basis to program the tooth movement directly on the bracket and not in wire bending, and were also the origin of the straight-wire, or preadjusted, appliance of current use in orthodontics. However, until now, the postulates of Andrews never have been contrasted using the scientific method and a proper statistical analysis. Moreover, some orthodontists have the suspect that the criteria of Andrews are not universal and applicable to the whole population since he do not distinguished age-dependent changes, ethnical group, sex, or left-right asymmetry. The critical analysis of the Andrews' work is the goal of this Chapter, but we have centered our efforts in the date related to Crown angulation (the mesiodistal "tip") and Crown inclination (labiolingual or buccolingual inclination) which are of capital importance to perform accurately functional and aesthetic orthodontic treatments.

2. Background: Historical context

The use of the fixed appliance in orthodontic is directly linked to the proposal and guides of Edward H. Angle to move the teeth to the so-called "occlusion line", defined as *"the line, shape and position, must be teeth in balance if there is a normal occlusion"*. Angle described in detail the relationships between maxillary and mandible, and maxillary-mandible and teeth, and especially the teeth among them, in order to achieve an ideal occlusion (Angle, 1929b; see the Special Edition of 1981).

These recommendations required the designing of special devices for three-dimensional control of teeth in order to reach the occlusion line and allow teeth to be correctly aligned in both the maxillary and mandible. Furthermore, according to Angle the alignment of the teeth, both crown and root, would result in the expansion of both the maxillary and mandible arches. This was also one of the main objectives to design the Angle's devices. Nevertheless, these postulates are still under discussion (Canut, 2000; Peck, 2008).

In 1887, Angle developed the "E" arch appliance formed by a thick gold wire placed for labial and some stainless steel tape on the first molar adjusted at pressure. This type of arch expanded both maxillary and mandible arches sagittally and transversely, and allowed a movement of simple inclination of the crown through a few ligatures that surrounded the tooth and conformed to the arch.

In the early 20th century with the development of metallurgy emerged the possibility of banding all the teeth and welding devices for the control of rotations. In 1910, Angle introduced the first appliance with individual tooth action and fullbanding, the so-called "pin and tube appliance", which welded small vertical tubes in the bands to introduce a stem attached to the wire. This device facilitated the labiolingual as mesiodistal expansion of the maxillary, and its drawback was the requirement for adjustment and accuracy in addition to the skill by the clinician (Bravo, 2007). Unfortunately one of the problems posed by this device was its inestability (Graber and Vanarsdall, 1994). Later, in 1916, Angle designed a bracket, called "ribbon arch appliance wire-band", containing a rectangular wire fixed by a few pins and placing the wider side on the tooth. This device properly controlled the labiolingual as well as vertical placement of teeth, by facilitating the correction of giroversions. However, it was difficult to place on the cusp and the looseness of the wire in the slot prevented mesiodistal control. Another substantial contribution of Angle was the frontal slot bracket, as opposed to the ribbon arch appliance of vertical opening, which featured great advantages, especially the ease to introduce the wire and the possibility to control the premolars and the adjustment of mesiodistal movement. In 1926 he presented the "bracket 447" with a horizontal slot .022 "x.028" which served to introduce a rectangular wire of the same thickness through the more narrow are, i.e. edgewise. It was made in gold and was called "soft bracket", as it opened easily and distorting (see for a review the Special Edition of Angle's work, 1981).

Over the basis of this model Steiner developed the "bracket 452" (hard bracket), more resistant to deformation which allowed to control teeth movement at the three levels through bends as tip, torque and in-out. This would become the prototype of the contemporary brackets.

Previously to the emergence of the straight wire, Angle already proposed to place the brackets to mesial or distal from the teeth to help to correct teeth rotations (Angle, 1929a), and a posterior angulation of the brackets to get proper root movements (see Meyer and Nelson, 1978). Later, Lewis (1950) joined segments ("arms") linked to the brackets, in contact with the wires for controlling rotations. Thereafter, Holdaway (1952) proposed that the buccal aspect of the brackets could be angulated depending on the degree of severity of the malocclusion. Twenty years later the original idea of Lewis, with some modifications, was adapted by Gottlieb et al. (1972). On the other hand Jarabak and Fizell (1963) minted the well-known phrase "building treatment into the appliance" which proposed to incorporate angles within the bracket, and these authors presented at the meeting of the American Association of Orthodontist in 1960 the first bracket model combining crown angulation and crown inclination (Wahl, 2008).

All together the work of all these authors consisted in eliminating bends in the wire to be incorporated into the bracket. All this led to the evolution of the bracket of edgewise to the bracket of straight wire incorporating the information in the slot of the bracket (Figure 1).

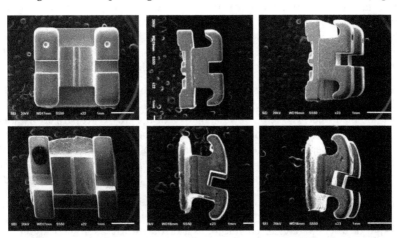

Fig. 1. Top line: Scanning electron microscopy of one bracket of standard edgewise appliance from a frontal (A), lateral (B), and oblique (C) view. Bottom line: Scanning electron microscopy of one straight wire bracket from a frontal (D), lateral (E), and oblique (F) view. The absence of information in the slot of the bracket of standard edgewise appliance in comparison with the bracket of the straight-wire appliance can be observed.

2.1 The work of L.F. Andrews

From 1960 Andrews published a series of five studies, which resulted in the development of a new concept for the orthodontic treatment: the straight wire appliance.

The **First study** had as purpose the completion of a thesis for obtaining the certification of the American Board of Orthodontics. It consisted of the static analysis of the occlusion in post-orthodontic treatment casts. He found that there were features common to all them: absence of rotations in the incisors, no cross-bites, and Class I molar relationship of Angle, except in cases of extractions in a single maxillary. However, other parameters were not common at all. He deduced that the optimal positioning of the teeth should sustain in studies of optimal natural dentures (see Andrews, 1989).

In order to perform the **Second study**, Andrews selected 120 casts of non-orthodontic, untreated, patients with supposedly ideal occlusions, from which arose a few assumptions that should determine the occlusal objectives after orthodontic treatment. The compilation of the cases was carried out between 1960 and 1964 with the help of various Orthodontists, among them Brodie (Andrews, 1989). These casts have in common, in addition to lack of orthodontic treatment, a correct teeth alignment and positioning as well as a seemingly an "excellent" occlusion. The concept was, in essence, that if it is know what is right it can identify and quantify what's wrong in a direct and methodical manner. Over the casts Andrews conducted a series of marks: the facial axis (axial) of the clinical crowns, the most prominent portion of incisors, canines and pre-molars, as well as the projection of the medial groove in molars, and the midpoint of the height of each clinical crown.

In the **Third study** he described six characteristics that were always present in the 120 casts. These features would be referred to as "*The six keys to normal occlusion*" and were published in 1972 in the American Journal of Orthodontics (Andrews, 1972). The "Six Keys" would assess the occlusal situation without using measuring instruments, as in the keys II and III (referring to the crown angulation and crown inclination, respectively), Andrews do not use units but simply the positive or negative sign (he used terms such as lightly positive, generally negative, etc). According to Andrews the "Six Keys" are interdependent components of the structural system of optimal occlusion and serve as a basis to assess the occlusion.

They consisted of a series of significant characteristics shared by all of the non-orthodontic normal teeth, and were the following: specific molar relationship (key I), crown angulation (the angulation or mesiodistal "tip" of the long axis of the crown: Key II), crown inclination (the labiolingual or buccolingual inclination of the long axis of the crown: Key III), no rotations (key IV), absence of spaces (key V), and the occlusal plane (key VI). In the own Andrews words "*The six keys to normal occlusion contribute individually and collectively to the total scheme of occlusion and, therefore, are viewed as essential to successful orthodontic treatment*".

The 120 casts analyzed by Andrews showed similarities in values of crown angulation, crown inclination, shape, and size for the different types of teeth. But this was not enough for the design of the new device. Therefore, in a further study attempted to determine the shape, size and position of each tooth in the arch.

For the **Fourth study**, Andrews made new measurements over the 120 casts (see Andrews, 1989). The measurements made in this case were: the determination of the bracket area for each teeth, vertical crown contour, crown angulation, crown inclination, offset of maxillary molars, horizontal crown contour, crown facial prominence and depth of the curve of Spee. So, he doubled the 120 casts and removed the occlusal halves of the crown. On these surfaces he defined a line that joins the portion more vestibular of contact points and the most prominent portions of each clinical crown. He denominated this line as the embrasure line. The values obtained were incorporated into the design of the bracket to eliminate the first order bends. These measurements, except bracket size and curve of Spee, were averaged for each tooth type, and the results served as norms for the design of the new appliance: the straight-wire. After describing outcomes, Andrews concludes that the study reveals essential data on the position (with the exception of the inclination of the incisors), morphology and relative vestibular prominence of each tooth in the arch. The differences in the inclination of the incisors were attributed to disharmonies between the maxillary bones.

The **Fifth**, and final, **study** consisted of comparison of 1156 casts post-treatment in terms of occlusion, with the 120 casts from non-treated subjects with optimal occlusion. This study was focused to the design of a new device able to include the "six keys". The conclusion was that very few of the analyzed casts presented all the "six keys" (Andrews, 1976a). Therefore, he considered necessary the establishment of some premises of treatment, including common objectives, coupled with a new device. The straight wire appliance of Andrews was the first completely pre-adjusted orthodontic appliance. It was designed for the treatment of cases without extraction with one less than 5° ANB, avoiding the need for bends in the wire. As the closure of the spaces after premolar extractions produces undesirable side effects (rotation, inclination), Andrews subsequently introduced different brackets for cases with extractions. Moreover, when designing their brackets, Andrews differentiated between treatments in which the translation of teeth is necessary and that no, the so-called brackets of translation and standard brackets (Andrews, 1976c, 1989). In a short time the new straight-wire appliance was adopted by the American universities and most of the orthodontists (Andrews, 1976b, 1989). Some year later (Roth, 1976, 1987), designed brackets with information at the three levels, varying the characteristics described by Andrews. He developed the second generation of preprogrammed brackets, increasing the crown inclination in the canines up to 13° to achieve the "best functional occlusion".

The third generation of brackets was developed by McLaughlin, Bennett and Trevisi (MBT™, McLaughlin et al., 1997; see also McLaughlin and Bennett, 1989). It is based on light forces and sliding mechanics maintaining the advantages of the prescriptions of Andrews and Roth, but eliminating certain limitations.

The introduction of straight-wire appliance in orthodontics led to a great controversy initially, but soon was accepted by all American orthodontic companies since it easily consent to control dental positions with the placement of brackets. Since then, others have developed new appliances, also fully programmed pre-adjusted (see for a review and references Proffit et al., 2008).

3. The Andrew's series: The values for crown angulation and crown inclination revisited

The first step of our work was to collect the individual values for crown angulation and crown inclination contained in the text and annex from Andrews' book "Straight-Wire, The Concept and Appliance" (Andrews, 1989), confirm that the descriptive statistical are exact, and apply to them a descriptive statistical analysis using the actual current methods.

When we try to validate the Andrews' statistical design the following questions and methodological troubles emerge when analyze the series of 120 casts that are the basis of the Andrews' work:

1. The origin of the sample: the author does not indicate how was selected the sample and what were the selection criteria;
2. The type of clustering of the data: he reports data from 240 casts instead of 120, because he evaluated together teeth from left and right side without checking whether or not there are differences between hemi-arch;
3. The variability between the data in the same group: the data are presented as a tabulation of centralization and dispersion of the maxillary and mandibular angles measures as did Andrews, with 240 data as if they were separate measures.

Therefore, our second step was the verification of the validity of the Andrew's design by contrast of hypothesis. It was carried out a Student t test of paired data to know whether or not there are significant differences in the crown angulation and crown inclination between the right and left hemi-arch with respect of their average values. The null hypothesis was that there are no significant differences in the crown angulation or crown inclination of teeth with respect to the side (p ≥ 0.05) and the study hypothesis was that there are significant differences in the crown angulation or crown inclination of teeth with respect to the side (p ≤ 0.05).

Descriptive statistics in the Andrew's series

Surprisingly, several errors in the basic descriptive statistics (count, average, standard deviation, minimum and maximum values) were detected for crown angulation but not for crown inclination (Tables 1 and 2). Thus, there is an error between the source (single) data and statistic results appearing in his publication. Moreover, in comparing these basic descriptive statistics with those obtained by us, applying the some probes on the Andrews data, it can be observed again that do not match for crown angulation (Table 1). Thus, there is an error between the source (single) data and statistic results appearing in his publication, and the statistics are no well calculated.

Tooth	Maxillary			Mandible		
	n	Range min/max	mean±SD	n	Range min/max	mean±SD
Andrews data/Our data						
1L+1R	240	-3/9	3.59±1.65	240	-4/3	0.53±1.29
1L+1R	240	-3/9	3.59±1.70	240	-4/3	0.53±1.29
2L+2R	240	**-2/15**	**8.04±2.80**	240	-5/3	0.38±1.47
2L+2R	240	-26/15	7.90±3.53	240	-5/3	0.38±1.48
3L+3R	239	**1/17**	**8.40±2.97**	240	-11/12	2.48±3.28
3L+3R	240	0/17	8.13±3.21	240	-11/12	2.48±3.29
4L+4R	240	**-2/12**	**2.65±1.69**	240	-10/10	1.28±1.90
4L+4R	240	-2/14	2.90±2.29	240	-10/10	1.28±1.90
5L+5R	240	0/12	**2.82±1.52**	240	-5/7	1.54±1.35
5L+5R	240	0/12	2.86±1.54	240	-5/7	1.54±1.36
6L+6R	240	-7/16	**5.73±1.90**	240	-2/6	2.03±1.14
6L+6R	240	-7/16	5.69±1.97	240	-2/6	2.03±1.14

Table 1. **Crown angulation.** Basic descriptive statistics of Andrews' data after revisited by us (black), and after the descriptive statistical study we have carried out (red). Values are expressed in degrees, and the observed differences are highlighted in bold.

Tooth	Maxillary			Mandible		
	n	Range min/max	mean±SD	n	Range min/max	mean±SD
Andrews data/Our data						
1L+1R	240	-7/15	6.11±3.97	240	-17/16	-1.71±5.79
1L+1R	240	-7/15	6.11±3.98	240	-17/16	-1.71±5.80
2L+2R	240	-6/17	4.42±4.38	239	-19/15	-3.24±5.37
2L+2R	240	-6/17	4,42±4.39	240	-19/15	-3.24±5.38
3L+3R	240	-17/10	-7.25±4.21	239	-26/2	-12.73±4.65
3L+3R	240	-17/10	-7.25±4.22	239	-26/2	-12.73±4.66
4L+4R	240	-20/5	-8.47±4.02	240	-35/-1	-18.95±4.96
4L+4R	240	-20/5	-8.47±4.03	239	-35/-1	-18.95±4.97
5L+5R	240	-20/3	-8.78±4.13	240	-45/-8	-23.63±5.58
5L+5R	240	-20/3	-8.78±4.14	240	-45/-8	-23.63±5.60
6L+6R	240	-25/2	-11.53±3.91	240	-55/-9	-30.67±5.90
6L+6R	240	-25/2	-11.53±3.92	240	-55/-9	-30.67±5.91

Table 2. **Crown inclination.** Basic descriptive statistics of Andrews' data after revisited by us (black), and after the descriptive statistical study we have carried out (red). Values are expressed in degrees, and the observed differences are highlighted in bold.

As Andrews considered the data together then we analyzed if there are differences between left and right teeth. For crown angulation, in comparing the average values of the right side and the left side differences were found to be significant (p<0.05) for all maxillary and mandibular teeth, except for the lower central incisor (Table 3). On the other hand, the comparison of mean averages for crown inclination of the right and left sides significant differences (p<0.05) were found for all upper teeth, except for the canines and first premolars, and for all lower teeth expect for both central and lateral incisors (Table 4).

Tooth	Maxillary			Mandible		
	t	fd	p	t	df	p value
1	3.00	119	**0.003**	1.11	119	0.270
2	5.71	119	**0.000**	-1.98	119	**0.050**
3	2.39	118	**0.013**	-2.62	119	**0.010**
4	2.30	119	**0.023**	-2.52	119	**0.013**
5	2.11	119	**0.037**	-3.86	119	**0.000**
6	2.79	119	**0.006**	-3.97	119	**0.000**

df: degrees of freedom

Table 3. **Crown angulation**. Student t test for crown angulation of right vs left arch. Significant differences are highlighted in bold.

Tooth	Maxillary			Mandible		
	t	fd	p	t	df	p values
1	4.00	119	**0.000**	0.11	119	0.909
2	4.95	119	**0.000**	-0.56	119	0.830
3	-1.22	119	0.223	-3.37	118	**0.008**
4	0.65	119	0.518	-4.60	118	**0.00**
5	2.34	119	**0.021**	-5.12	119	**0.000**
6	2.99	119	**0.003**	-6.56	119	**0.000**

df: degrees of freedom

Table 4. **Crown inclination**. Student t test for crown inclination for right vs left arch. Significant differences are highlighted in bold.

These results consent to affirm that significant differences exists between the right and left sides of each arch, for the angulation of crown for all the teeth of the upper arch, and for the majority of the lower arch. Regarding the crown inclination significant differences do not occur in all the maxillary and mandibular teeth but all show any difference.

3.1 Descriptive statistics of separate hemi-arch

Since significant differences between the right and left hemi-arch were found in the Andrews' series we decided to perform and basic descriptive statistical analysis of both crown angulation and crown inclination in each hemi-arch separately. At a value of the confidence interval 95% the standard deviation shows very high values in some teeth, and the variable dispersion is therefore very broad.

In the upper maxillary the greater homogeneity in crown angulation was found for the central incisor, the second premolar and first molar (Table 5; Fig. 2A). The mandible crown angulation shows a more homogeneous behavior, except for the canine (Table 5; Fig. 2B). The presence of outlier values implies a high variability, and so at a confidence interval 95% wider than would be desirable (Figs. 3A and 3C, and Figs. 3B and 3D).

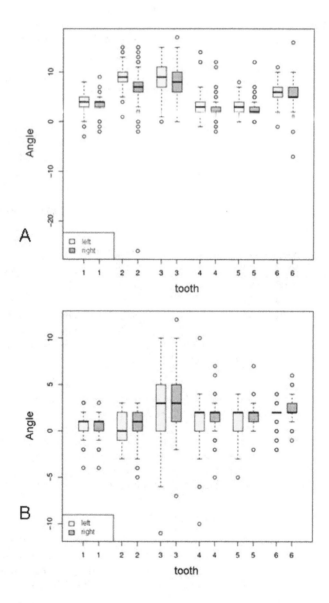

Fig. 2. Box-plot representation of the maxillary crown angulation (A) and mandibular crown angulation (B) of the data from the Andrews' series.

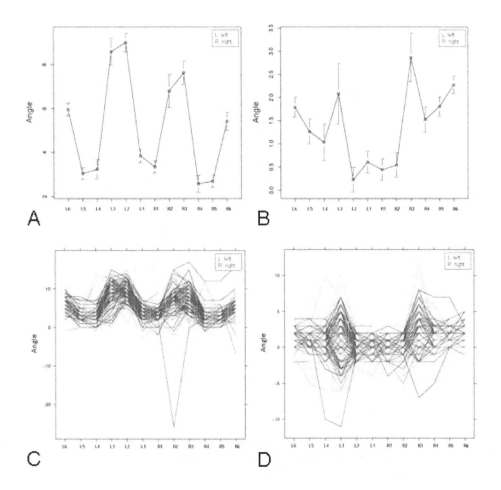

Fig. 3. Mean values of confidence interval 95% and profiles of the maxillary crown angulation (A,C) and mandibular crown angulation (B,D) of the data from the Andrews' series.

Tooth		n	mean±SD	range of confidence interval
Right hemi-arch				
1R	upper	120	3.42±1.56	3.06 - 3.62
	lower	120	0.44±1.28	0.21 - 0.67
2R	upper	120	6.79±2.85	6.04 - 7.54
	lower	120	0.54±1.46	0.28 - 0.81
3R	upper	119	7.61±2.93	7.07 - 8.16
	lower	120	2.87±2.89	2.34 - 3.39
4R	upper	120	2.57±2.13	2.19 - 2.96
	lower	120	1.52±1.51	1.25 - 1.80
5R	upper	120	2.69±1.55	2.40 - 2.98
	lower	120	1.81±1.13	1.60 - 2.01
6R	upper	120	5.42±2.12	5.01 - 5.82
	lower	120	2.27±1.04	2.09 - 2.46
Left hemi-arch				
1R	upper	120	3.84±1.70	3.53 - 4.15
	lower	120	0.61±1.30	0.37 - 0.84
2R	upper	120	9.00±2.33	8.58 - 9.42
	lower	120	0.54±1.48	0.28 - 0.81
3R	upper	120	8.58±3.37	7.97 - 9.20
	lower	120	2.87±3.61	2.34 - 3.39
4R	upper	120	3.23±2.43	2.80 - 3.67
	lower	120	1.52±2.20	1.25 - 1.80
5R	upper	120	3.03±1.47	2.77 - 3.30
	lower	120	1.81±1.50	1.60 - 2.01
6R	upper	120	5.96±1.62	5.66 - 6.25
	lower	120	2.27±1.19	2.09 - 2.46

Table 5. **Crown angulation.** Basic descriptive statistics of Andrews' data for hemi-arch after revisited by us. Values are expressed in degrees.

The results for crown inclination are reflected in table 6, and Figures 4A and 4B, which show that the variability of the data is very similar for all teeth. The mandible data presented a top-down performance in terms of average values of the central incisor to the first molar. The study of confidence intervals 95% shows differences between the teeth and the side. In general, the profiles of the subjects were similar for both the maxillary and mandibular teeth (Figs. 5A and 5C, and Figs. 5B and 5D).

Are the Orthodontic Basis Wrong? Revisiting Two of the Keys to Normal Oclusion (Crown Inclination and Crown Angulation) in the Andrews Series

39

Tooth		n	mean±SD	range of confidence interval
Right hemi-arch				
1R	upper	120	5.76±4.01	-2.76 – -0.67
	lower	120	-1.71±5.77	0.21 – 0.67
2R	upper	120	3.83±4.43	3.03 – 4.63
	lower	120	-3.25±5.60	-4.26 – -2.24
3R	upper	120	-7.02±4.52	-7.84 – -6.21
	lower	119	-12.19±4.28	-12.96 – -11.42
4R	upper	120	-8.57±4.11	-9.31 – -7.82
	lower	119	-18.12±4.95	-19.01 – -17.22
5R	upper	120	-9.17±4.23	-9.93 – -8.40
	lower	120	-22.49±5.46	-23.48 – -21.50
6R	upper	120	-12.0±4.08	-12.73 – -11.26
	lower	120	-29.4±5.75	-30.44 – -28.36
Left hemi-arch				
1R	upper	120	6.47±3.94	5.75 – 7.18
	lower	120	-1.70±5.85	-2.76 – -0.64
2R	upper	120	5.00±4.28	4.23 – 5.77
	lower	120	-3.21±5.15	-4.14 – -2.28
3R	upper	120	-7.47±3.90	-8.17 – -6.76
	lower	120	-13.17±5.01	-14.09 – -12.24
4R	upper	120	-8.37±3.96	-9.09 – -7.66
	lower	120	-19.78±4.87	-20.66 – -18.90
5R	upper	120	-8.39±4.01	-9.12 – -7.66
	lower	120	-24.77±5.81	-25.76 – -23.77
6R	upper	120	-11.07±3.71	-11.74 – -10.39
	lower	120	-31.93±8.02	-32.98 – -30.88

Table 6. **Crown inclination.** Basic descriptive statistics of Andrews' data for hemi-arch after revisited by us. Values are expressed in degrees.

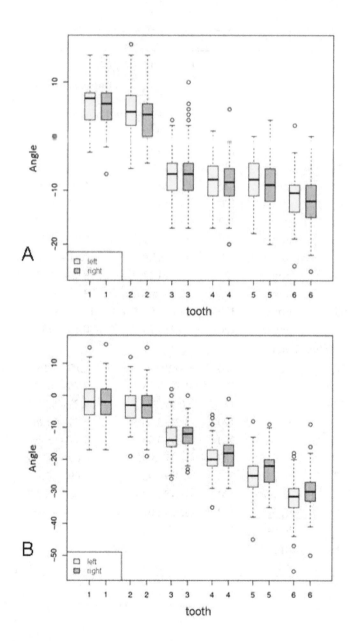

Fig. 4. Box-plot representation of the maxillary crown inclination (A) and mandibular crown inclination (B) of the data from the Andrews' series.

Are the Orthodontic Basis Wrong? Revisiting Two of the Keys to Normal Oclusion (Crown Inclination and Crown Angulation) in the Andrews Series

41

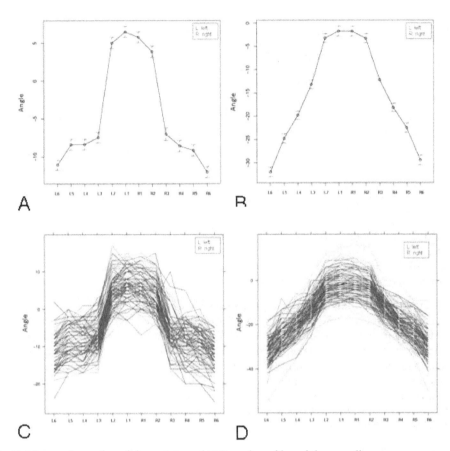

Fig. 5. Mean values of confidence interval 95% and profiles of the maxillary crown inclination (A,C) and mandibular crown inclination (B,D) of the data from the Andrews' series.

3.2 Critical comments to the Andrews' work

After the analysis of the data published by Andrews (1989) in his book *Straight-Wire, The Concept and Appliance* the first thing that draws attention is that the author annex provide data relating to 240 casts instead of 120, which are those said to have studied. This may be due to the fact that the author carried out two measurements by subject (left and right) in each arch, and then globalize the data into a single; but Andrews does not clarify this fact. Is this right? The statistical study we have performed on the Andrews' data shows that there are significant differences between left and right for crown angulation and crown inclination for most of the upper teeth, and form the lower teeth for crown angulation of the lateral incisor to the first molar, and for crown inclination in the canine, premolars and first molar. Therefore, it seems evident that the data from the Andrews study cannot be grouped, and it is necessary to work with each hemi-arch separately and perform the descriptive and comparative analysis for each one of them. From these results the following question arises: it should be necessary use different brackets on left and right side of each patient?

Another surprising finding of our review of the Andrews' data was that the results presented in terms of basic descriptive statistic not always coincide with those from the sources. These errors can be due to erroneous data sheets records or that have been made evil the descriptive analysis.

The Andrews' results are expressed as average values, and the standard deviation was occasionally elevated, thus reflecting a significant dispersion of the sample values. For example, the following measurements for crown angulation (mean±standard deviation, range; minimal-maximal) in the first premolar realize this: upper $2.65°\pm1.69°$, $-2.0°$ to $+12°$; lower: $2.90°\pm2.29°$, $-2°$ to $+14°$. The ranges show the enormous variation of values. If in cases of optimal occlusions the crown angulation of this tooth vary between $-2°$ and $12°$, take as reference a value of $2.65°$ in orthodontic appliances does not seems logical.

It would also be desirable that Andrews had studied the type of the data distribution in the sample, and the author seems to assume that the distribution is symmetric, but in the light of the results presented here, it is unlikely to be so. In fact, the normality test indicates that the distribution is not normal in all cases.

The listing of all the individual data of the sample is a sign of honesty by the author, and reflects the statistical methodology of the 1970s. But at the same time it allows us to appreciate their low methodological rigor, in the light of current knowledge when presenting the conclusions as a definitive response to a widely discussed problem. Thus, it is difficult to understand why the orthodontists from around the world have continued to put the brackets using as a reference the average values of the measurements made on 120 casts without rigorous selection criteria. In our casts, as well as in those from other groups (Roth, 1987; Martínez-Asúnsolo and Plasencia, 2004; Zanelato et al., 2004), the findings of Andrews for the crown angulation and inclinations were not confirmed.

Therefore, the Andrews study in terms of design, include the following shortcomings: definition of the characteristics of the sample, the exact criteria of selection of the subjects included in the sample, the absence of a descriptive statistic that analyze the way of the distribution of the data (if distribution is markedly asymmetrical, would be preferable to choose the mean than the average as a measure of central tendency), the type of sampling, and sample size calculation. In the Andrews study the sample size is adequate (240 measurements from 120 casts). Nevertheless, to work with greater precision, for example 0.5 mm, the sample should be higher.

On the other hand, the development of the work of Andrews also suffers from some defects. In this kind of studies it is necessary to assess their reproducibility or reliability, both intra-observer and inter-observed. It is not aware that the Andrews work has been performed by several observers, and therefore it must be we assumed that the measurements were carried out by Andrews himself or by another individual. Still, in any case Andrews should be repeated, at least once more, all measures in the same models and to analyze the reliability between measurements. Also, as quantitative variables, the degree of reliability should have been studied through the appropriate statistical tests: Bradley-Blackwood, correlation coefficient, tor the Student t test for paired samples. The errors we have detected in the

Are the Orthodontic Basis Wrong? Revisiting Two of the Keys to Normal Oclusion (Crown Inclination and Crown Angulation) in the Andrews Series

43

Andrews work are surely sufficient to raise necessary a reassessment of the theories of the straight wire. The real debate must be focused on whether the recommendations of Andrews for the crown angulation an inclination may continue to be used for the creation, development and industrialization of orthodontic appliances to serve for the entire population. The tooth size (Agenter et al., 2009; Lee et al., 2011), the place of each teeth in each side hemi-arch, the gender, and the ethnic group (Naranjilla and Rudzki-Janson, 2005) should be considered in the development of future orthodontic appliances.

4. Concluding remarks

While Andrews work is thorough and interesting for its time, it has enough limitations of design or execution to be considered actually as the foundations for the use of an appliance with universal angulation and inclination. Furthermore, we have not found one sufficient material and methodology description in the of Andrews' work to reproduce it accurately. In fact a number of errors in the results of basic descriptive statistics were detected in the Andrews' series. This could be due to errors is the data sheet, or to errors in calculating descriptive statistics.

On the other hand, it cannot be included in a common sample data from measurements obtained from the right and left sides of the maxillary and the mandible as Andrews, given that there are significant differences between the average values of both sides. Therefore it does not seem appropriate to use average angle and tilt values without specifying the side of the arch which belongs to the tooth. Considering the large standard deviations observed in values from the Andrews' series the values of both inclination and angulation cannot be standardized. The variations in the values of angulation and inclination reported by different authors would be sufficient to raise the need for a re-evaluation of the theories of the straight-wire appliance in orthodontics.

5. References

Agenter MK, Harris EF, Blair RN. 2009. Influence of tooth crown size on malocclusion. Am J Orthod Dentofacial Orthop 136:795-804.

Andrews LF. 1972. The six keys to normal occlusion. Am J Orthod 62: 296-309.

Andrews LF. 1976a. The diagnostic system: occlusal analysis. Dent Clin North Am 20:671-690.

Andrews LF. 1976b. The straight-wire appliance archform, wire bending & an experiment. J Clin Orthod. 10:581-588.

Andrews. LF. 1976c. The straight-wire appliance. Extraction brackets and classification of treatment. J Clin Orthod 10:360-377.

Andrews LF. 1989. Straight Wire. The concept and appliance. San Diego, L.A.: Wells Company.

Angle EH. 1929a. The latest and best in orthodontic mechanism. Dental Cosmos 71: 164-173.

Angle EH. 1929b. The latest and best in orthodontic mechanism. Dental Cosmos 71:260-720.

Angle EH. 1981. Treatment of malocclusion of the teeth. Special Edition. Ed. The Classics of Dentistry Library. Birmingham Alabama Division of Gryphon Editions Ltd., pp. 198-262.

Bravo LA. 2007. Manual de Ortodoncia. Madrid Ed. Síntesis S.A., pp. 372-375. (Spanish text)

Canut JA. 2000. Ortodoncia clínica y terapéutica. 2ª edición. 2000. Barcelona Ed. Masson S.A., pp. 18-21. (Spanish text)

Gottlieb EL, Wildman AJ, Lang HM, Lee IF, Struch EC Jr. 1972. The Edgelok bracket. J Clin Orthod 6:613-623.

Graber TM, Vanarsdall RL Jr. 1994. Orthodontics Currents Principles and Techniques. 2ª edición. St. Louis, Missouri. Ed Mosby-YearBook Inc., pp. 627-635.

Holdaway RA. 1952. Bracket angulation as applied to the edgewise appliance. Angle Orthod 22:227-236.

Jarabak JR, Fizell JA. 1963. Technique and treatment with the light-wire appliance. Sant Louis, Missouri. Mosby.

Lee GJ, Ahn SJ, Lim WH, Lee S, Lim J, Park HJ. 2011. Variation of the intermaxillary tooth-size relationship in normal occlusion. Eur J Orthod 33:9 14.

Lewis PD. 1950. Space closure in extraction cases. Am J Orthod 36: 172-191.

McLaughlin RP, Bennett JC. 1989. The transition from standard edgewise to preadjusted appliance systems. J Clin Orthod 23:142-153.

McLaughlin R, Bennett J, Trevisi H. 1997. A clinical review of the MBT orthodontic treatment program. Orthod Perspec 4:3-15.

Martinez-Asúnsolo P, Plasencia E. 2004. Las 6 llaves de la oclusión de Andrews en 32 modelos con oclusiones ideales no tratadas. Rev Esp Ortod 34:235-244 (Spanish text)

Meyer M, Nelson G. 1978. Preajusted edgewise appliances: Theory and practice. Am J Orthod 73:485-498.

Naranjilla MA, Rudzki-Janson I. 2005. Cephalometric features of fi lipinos with class I occlusion according to the Munich analysis. Angle Orthod 75:63-68.

Peck S. 2008. So what's new? Arch expansion again. Angle Orthod 78:574-575.

Proffitt WR, Fields HW, Sarver DM. 2008. Ortodoncia Contemporánea. 4ª edición. Elsevier España 2008 Barcelona (Spanish Edition)

Roth RH. 1976. Five year clinical evaluation of the Andrews straight-wire appliance. J Clin Orthod 10:836-850.

Roth RH. 1987. The straight-wire appliance 17 years later. J Clin Orthod 21:632-642.

Wahl N. 2008. Orthodontics in 3 millenia. Chapter 16: Late 20th-century fixed appliances. Am J Orthod Dentofacial Orthop 134: 827-830.

Zanelato RC, Grossi AT, Mandetta S. 2004. Individualización de torque para los caninos en aparatos preajustados. Rev Ortodon Dental Press 3:39-55.

3

The Importance and Possibilities of Proper Oral Hygiene in Orthodontic Patients

Melinda Madléna
Semmelweis University
Hungary

1. Introduction

The number of orthodontic treatments has been increased nowdays (Silva & Kang, 2001; Thilander et al., 2001; Ciuffolo et al., 2005; Mtaya et al, 2009; Bittencourt & Machado, 2010). The most important motivation for orthodontic treatment is to achieve an improvement in appearance and the fact that in connection with this change some psychological problems could be decreased. These factors are contributed not only to the position but the esthetic appearance of the tooth itself. In some cases orthodontic treatments can attribute to caries preventive intervention, when tooth movements may reduce crowding or other anomalies, thus can contribute to the effectiveness of proper oral hygiene. On the other hand, orthodontic treatments may cause or aggravate plaque accumulation and in this way the development of caries and periodontal diseases which are basically caused by dental plaque. It is suggested that the information about both benefits and risks of orthodontic treatment should be sheared with potential patients.

This chapter explaines the relationships between orthodontic anomalies and orthodontic treatments and dental plaque induced diseases, delineates how to determinate the risk of the orthodontic treatment causing dental caries and periodontal diseases. The third part of this chapter summarizes the possibilities to avoid and reduce these effects using different modern equipments, techniques and adjuvants.

2. Relations between orthodontic anomalies / orthodontic treatment and dental plaque induced diseases

2.1 Associations of the orthodontic anomalies with dental caries

It is wellknown for a long time that in some orthodontic cases patients have greater difficulties in maintaining proper oral hygiene (Katz, 1978; Miller & Hobson, 1961). In spite of this, some authors published no correlation between positional anomalies and the caries prevalence. Helm and Petersen (1989a) examined 176 adolescents aged 13-19 years and re-examined them after 20 years in order to detect any relationship between malocclusion and caries, found no association between malocclusion traits and caries prevalence. Other authors published the relationship between the dental caries and the presence of certain malocclusions concerning oral hygiene (e.g. crowding) (Gábris et al., 2006; Nobile et al., 2007; Mtaya et al, 2009). Stahl & Grabowski (2004) reported no positive correlation between prevalence of caries and any malocclusion in primary teeth but in their study significant parallelism in prevalence of malocclusion and caries was found for posterior cross-bite and mandibular overjet in children with mixed dentition.

2.2 Associations of the orthodontic anomalies with periodontal parameters concerning oral hygiene

The accumulation of plaque can cause gingival redness, bleeding, edema, changes in gingival morphology, reduced tissue adaptation to the teeth, an increase in the flow of gingival crevicular fluid and other clinical signs of inflammation (Figure 1). Maloccluded teeth can be associated with periodontal diseases because of the physically hampered proper oral hygiene.

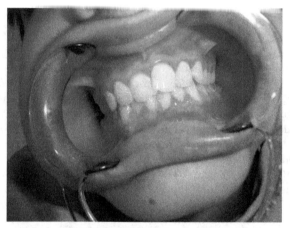

Fig. 1. Crowded frontal teeth with large amount of plaque.

In case of this anomaly the oral hygiene is harmful, the plaque elimination needs more time and special method. The picture shows a gingivitis as a consequence of the lack of proper oral hygiene.

According to the oral hygiene the most important basic symptom which can show more serious periodontal problems is gingival bleeding on probing (Geiger, 2001). The presence of a positive correlation between malocclusion (e.g. crowding, when the removal of plaque is difficult) and periodontal health has been described by Helm and Petersen (1989b) and Gábris et al. (2006), but on the contrary other studies found no association between amount of plaque or periodontal parameters and malocclusion (including crowding and spacing) (Geiger et al., 1974; Katz, 1978; Buckley, 1980). Other results had been published by Geiger (2001) found the possible associations between certain malocclusions (eg. anterior overjet and overbite, crossbite etc.) and periodontal problems, but these cases probably are not really in connection with oral hygiene.

2.3 Plaque accumulation concerning removable and fixed orthodontic appliances

The great plaque accumulation on different dental materials has been wellknown for a long time. From these points of view, we also consider removable appliances. In case of removable appliances, the resin base has microporosity. The greater accumulation of plaque on dental materials than on natural enamel is also wellknown (Skjörland, 1973). This is an increase in microorganisms which can provide an increased risk of carious lesions theoretically. Thus basically the orthodontic treatment with removable appliance causes an additional problem for the oral environment. The surface of the removable appliance will be coated within a short time mainly with streptococci and gram negative and positive rods (Bickel & Geering, 1982). According to the results of Batoni et al. (2001) the use of removable appliances may lead to the creation of new retentive areas and surfaces, which favour the local adherence and growths of streptococcus mutans. However, Schlagenhauf et al. (1989) found that the increase in number of streptococcus mutans was not significant in patients having removable orthodontic appliance comparing to those who weared fixed appliance.

The plaque accumulation is promoted by the physical constituton of different parts of fixed appliance, but there are some other factors having a great importance on plaque accumulation. In the oral cavity all of the tooth surfaces are exposed and rapidly covered by salivary proteins causing different effects (interactions between material, pellicle and bacteria). As a part of fixed appliances, orthodontic bands can cause a gingiva inflammation (Huser et al., 1990). Plaque accumulates particularly beneath bands from which some cement has been washed out adjacent to adhesive retention elements (Gwinnett & Cheen, 1979; Mizrahi, 1982). Plaque is found predominantly cervically to brackets under the arch wires. The scores of different periodontal parameters (Plaque Index, Gingival Bleeding Index) and proportion of spirochetes were found higher for banded molars than for molars with brackets (Boyd & Baumrind, 1992; Freundorfer et al. 1993). The loss of attachment is the highest approximally, particularly in adults, because the margins of band are frequently located subgingivally at approximal sites. In this way band with subgingival margins can promote the higher accumulation of the amount of plaque and contribute to development of gingivitis or periodontitis. In case of periodontitis besides the inflammation of gingiva the loss of connective tissue attachment (wich is irreversible change) also can be seen in the periodontium. In these situations gram negative and anaerobic microrganisms (Porphyromonas gingivalis, Prevotella intermedia, Actinomyces) are disproportionally present along the subgingival band margins (Diamanti-Kpioti et al., 1987) which are frequently associated with further periodontal problems. Beside of this, there is an increased number of spirochetes, mobile rods and fusiform organisms. Gingival hyperplasia may also occure and this complicates the oral hygiene and the dental treatment procedures (Figure 2.)

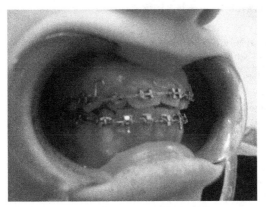

Fig. 2. Gingival hyperplasia in patient undergoing orthodontic treatment with fixed appliance.

The situation is caused by neglected oral hygiene, which complicate the treatment and oral hygienic procedures.

It has ben published that the elements of fixed orthodontic appliance can change the biologic balance in the oral cavity (Figure 3.).

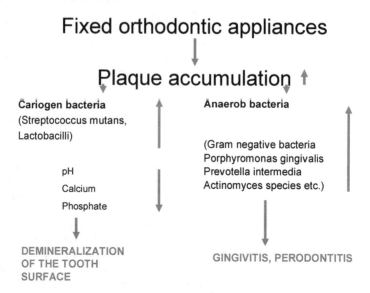

Fig. 3. Risk of treatment with fixed orthodontic appliances.

Plaque in patients with fixed orthodontic appliance has a lower pH than in non-orthodontic patients (Gwinnett & Cheen, 1979). There is a rapid shift in the composition of the bacterial flora, especially there is an increase in the levels of acidogenic bacteria (streptococcus mutans, lactobacilli), which leads to a decrease in pH. As the pH drop reaches the level of critical value (pH 5.5), the demineralization-remineralization balance is pushed toward mineral loss and demineralization/decalcification.

2.3.1 Decalcification of enamel caused by dental plaque accumulation (white spot lesions) during orthodontic treatment with fixed appliances

The first clinical evidence of the demineralization is the white spot lesion (WSL), which potentially can become a cavitated carious lesion extending even into the dentin (Featherstone, 2003; Featherstone et al, 2007). White spot lesions are nonfluoridated opacities having a more defined shape and are well differentiated from sorrounding enamel which are often located in the middle of the tooth (Sangamesh & Amitabh, 2011). The WSL has been defined as „subsurface enamel porosity from carious demineralization" presenting itself as a „milky white opacity" when located on smooth surfaces (Nicholson, 2006). Beside of that fact that WSL is a first step to destruction of the teeth, this enamel demineralization associated with fixed orthodontic appliances means an other significant clinical problem for the orthodontists (Ogaard, 1989; Bishara & Ostby, 20008). Because of the plaque accumulation on typical places, without proper oral hygiene, during or after the orthodontic treatment demineralization (white spot lesions) can be observed at these above mentioned plaque retention sites and the location of possible carious lesions are changed compared to the situation without orthodontic appliances (Muhler, 1970). The white spot lesions are predominantly appeare on the lower and upper premolars, first molars, maxillary and mandibular lateral inciors and lower canines as a change of tooth structure around the brackets basis or between the brackets/bands and gingival margin in the cervical region and middle third of the teeth, under the orthodontic wires (Ogaard, 2008). The frequency of WSL in orthodontically treated patients were in order lateral incisors, canines, first premolars, 2nd premolars, central incisors (Ogaard, 1989; Chapman et al., 2010). An other previous study showed similar results except those finding that the maxillary central incisors had a greater frequency of WSLs than did the maxillary second premolars (Gorelick et al., 1982). No significant differences were found in WSL incidence and prevalence between the right and left sides of the maxilla and mandible (Gorelick et al., 1982; Ogaard, 1989).

Evaluation of white spot lesions can be performed by macroscopic methods (clinical examination, photographic examination, optical nonfluorescent and fluorescent methods), microscopic methods (orthodontic caries models) and research methods (assessing different preventive agents) (Benson, 2008). The detected prevalence depends on the analytic methods. The highest prevalence of demineralization was detected by quantitative light induced fluorescence method which is much more sensitive than the simple direct visualization (Boersma, 2005). Inspector's unique analysis software is available to determinate the demineralization (Amaechi, 2009). Sound tooth tissue will show up glowing brightly without reflections, demineralised areas generally have a diffuse outline and are darker at the center which distinguishes them from stains and discoloration.

According to the study of Gorelick et al. (1982) the incidence of white spot formation in patients treated with fixed orthodontic appliances was nearly 50% compared to 24% in an untreated control group. In the literature great variations have been published (from 2 - to 97% of the patients) for WSL prevalence associated with orthodontic treatment (Zachrisson and Zachrisson, 1971; Gorelick et al., 1982; Mizrahi, 1982; Artun & Brobakken, 1986; Geiger et al., 1988; Ogaard, 1989; Mitchell, 1992). Although orthodontic patients had significantly more WSLs than non-orthodontic patients but in this stage generally were not registered as caries, requiring restorative treatment (Ogaard et al., 2004). However in some cases, the development of these lesions could be such rapid that it requiers rapid debonding and treatment procedures. It can be occured already within 4 weeks (Ogaard et al., 1988). Carious lesions may appear after debonding in association with bonded retainer also. Earlier studies showed increased caries frequency and higher prevalence of caries and also fillings in persons treated with fixed orthodontic appliances, but most of the further investigations did not confirm this statement which could be in connection with the higher motivation of the patients and the widespread possibility of oral hygiene regimens (Ingerwall, 1962; Zachrisson & Zachrisson, 1971; Hollender & Ronnerman, 1978; Southard et al., 1986; Ogaard, 1989). Muhler (1970) published that the orthodontic treatment without proper oral prophylaxis resulted in an increased incidence of caries which was significantly reduced after an appropriate prophylaxis. According to the study of Zachrisson & Zachrisson (1971) in case of cooperative patients with proper oral hygiene dental caries is a relatively minor problem and the number of new cavities is relatively low but it is contributed by different factors. For example, beside of the individual susceptibility, it has to be considered that generally the patients aged 6-10 years and during an early period of adolescents are in active caries phase, the number of new cavities may increase rapidly during fixed orthodontic treatment in these cases. The publicated incidence and prevalence of WSL can vary by sex. Although Ogaard (1989) found no significant difference between genders, most of the studies published it. According to the study of Zachrisson & Zachrisson (1971), girls had better caries index scores, (and also better periodontal indices) than boys during orthodontic treatment. In spite of these findings, Gorelick et al. (1982) found that females have higher incidence in WSL prevalence, while Boersma (2005) and Al Maaltah et al. (2011) published higher incidence of WSL in male. Chapmen et al. (2010) published a higher incidence of WSLs and also the more severe demineralization in males compared with female patients. It can be in connection with those results of some authors that female patients have been shown to have a greater interest in oral health, they had better oral health and tend to brush and floss their tooth more frequently (Kuusela et al., 1996; Sakki et al., 1998; Ostberg et al., 1999). Chapmen et al. (2010) published that early age at start of fixed appliance treatment, inadequate oral hygiene before the treatment, many treatment appointments with poor oral hygiene were associated with greater incidence and severity of WSLs. Al Maaltah et al. (2011) published that patients with WSLs were significantly younger and more likely to have diseased first molars.

Classification of white spot lesions can be found in a modification of material in publication of Nyvad et al. (1999):

White spot stage 1. Inactive caries (intact surface):

Surface of enamel is white, brown or black. It is glossy with no loss of luster; feels smooth and hard when the tip of the probe is gently moved across the surface. No clinically detectable loss of enamel. Smooth surface lesion typically located away from the gingival margin.

White spot stage 2. Inactive caries (surface discontinuity):

Surface enamel is white, brown or black. It is glossy with no loss of luster; feels smooth and hard when the tip of the probe is gently moved across the surface. Localized surface defects (microcavity) could be found in enamel only. No undermined enamel or softened floor detectable with the explorer.

When on the surface there are cavitated lesion, enamel/dentin cavity easily visible with naked eye, surface cavity feels hard on gentle probing and appears shiney. There is no pulpal involvement.

3. Determination of the risk causing dental caries and periodontal diseases during orthodontic treatment

It is wellknown that because of the great possibility for the increased plaque accumulation orthodontic patients who are treated with fixed appliance, mainly generally belong to a potentially higher risk group. So a list of risk factors should be recorded for orthodontic patients to identify those persons who need special preventive interventions. Orthodontic treatment may be hazardous for those patients who have no motivaton, no proper supervision or preventive programme. To notice the increased plaque accumulation, it is important for both patients and clinicians to prevent tooth decay, gingival or periodontal problems and tooth discoloration that could compromise the esthetic of smile and well being of the patients. The key for this is represented by dental plaque.

3.1 Identification of dental plaque

Dental plaque is „the soft tenaciosus material found on tooth surfaces which is not readily removed by rinsing with water" (Axelsson, 2000) (Figure 4.).

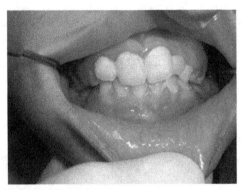

Fig. 4. Unstained dental plaque on the labial dental surfaces, on the cervical regions of the frontal teeth.

In this patient the consequences of the large amount of plaque (decalcification, gingivitis) are also seen.

In some cases the identification of plaque can be hard with the naked eye because it could have a whitish colour, similarly to the teeth. The plaque amount and localization can be determined by different methods. The simpliest way to scrape the tooth surface with a periodontal probe. Special test tablets containing red or blue dye can be used to stain the plaque. One tablet is chewed thoroughly, moving the mixture of saliva and dye over the teeth and gums for approximately 30 seconds. Then the mouth is rinsed with water and teeth are checked to identify the stained unremoved plaque. The disadvantage of these tablets that may cause a temporary pink or blue color of lips, cheeks, mouth or tongue. (Figure 5.). An other method is using plaque fluorescence. A special fluorescent solution is swirled around the mouth. After that the mouth is rinsed gently with water and the teeth and gums can be checked with an ultraviolet light. The plaque will be coloured in a brillant orange-yellow. This method does not leave stains on other tissues in the mouth.

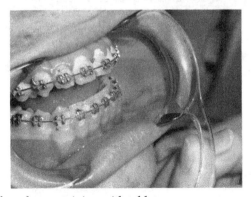

Fig. 5. The situation after plaque staining with tablets.

The method cause a temporary discoloration on the bucca or the tongue. Matured and fresh plaque can be seen in different colors. More blue plaque coloration means inproper oral hygiene

Some types of plaque staining products can differentiate between the cariogenic and noncariogenic plaque with different colors (Figure 5.). Acid producing ability of a plaque sample and its cariogenic potential can be determined. Non-cariogenic samples turn green or yellow, while cariogenic plaque samples turn red or orange after sucrose challenge from the solution. Some products contain a neutralising solution (e.g. Plaque Indicator Kit from the GC) which can be used for education of the patients, eg. regarding the protective actions of the saliva and a disclosing gel for the demonstration of plaque. The composition of plaque changes in time, which allows pathogenic bacteria to be active on the tooth surface. Using a special disclosing gel, a more than 48 hours old (matured) plaque and a fresh plaque can be seen in two different colours (blue, redish-pink).

The Inspektor QLF-D BiLuminator™ is a sophisticated device for assessment and monitoring of oral hygiene in the dental surgery. The QLF-D BiLuminator software supports easy acquisition of image pairs and orders them automatically on a visit-patient basis. Plaque and calculus show up brightly red in the QLF –image made by this equipment (Figure 6.). Only those plaque will be seen that has been present for some time (> 1 day).

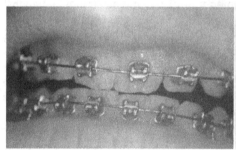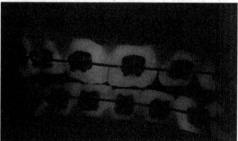

Fig. 6. White light and QLF image of teeth with orthodontic brackets (publication of the pictures with permission of Inspektor Research System BV, Netherlands).

The BiLuminator™ can be tremendous help to prevent any damage that may follow the placement of orthodontic brackets. By regularly inspecting teeth it can be ensured that teeth are well cleaned before the brackets are placed and mature plaque will not seen during the orthodontic treatment (Amaechi, 2009).

3.1.1 Measurement of plaque amount

There are a lot indices for the measurement of plaque amount, among them the index of Silness and Löe (1964) which is very easy to use, is one of the most frequently used in clinical practice. The Plaque Accumulation Rate Index (PFRI) performed by Axelsson (1991), based on the amount of disclosed plaque which is freely accumulated in the 24 hours following professional mechanical tooth cleaning (during which period subjects refrain from all oral hygiene practices. For the PFRI a five point scale was constructed (Figure 7.). There are positive correlations between the scores of PFRI and e.g. gingival bleeding, Plaque Index, level of streptococcus mutans, caries prevalence etc. (Axelsson, 2000).

Plaque Formation Rate Index
(PFRI) (Axelsson, 1991)

- **Score 1**: 1 to 10% of surfaces affected: very low
- **Score 2**: 11 to 20% of surfaces affected: low
- **Score 3**: 21 to 30% of surfaces affected: moderate
- **Score 4**: 31 to 40% of surfaces affected: high
- **Score 5**: more than 40% of surfaces affected: very high

Fig. 7. The scores of Plaque Formation Rate Index by Axelsson (1991).

3.2 Microbiological and clinical parameters for determination of caries risk

As caries is a multicausal disease, it is not optimal to examine just one etiological factor for the general prognosis. Caries risk assessment models involve a combination of factors including diet, fluoride exposure, a susceptible host, microflora which all can interplay with a variety of social, cultural and behavioural factors (Featherstone, 2003; Nicolau et al., 2003).

The combination of clinical and microbiological findings increases the sensitivity of caries prognosis to almost 100% (Kneist et al., 1998; Krasse, 1988). New carious lesions will develop if high bacterial counts have been recorded, thus the evaluation of microbiological data is also recommended before the starting of orthodontic treatment, because the caries risk tends to increase dramatically in patients with high bacterial counts after the placement of brackets, due to the difficulties in performing adequate oral hygiene (Kristofferson et al., 1985).

The risk of caries can be determined by other different testing procedures, these are based on determination of quality and quantity of saliva.

3.2.1 Microbiological parameters

In a regular dental practice the „chairside tests" are very easy to apply for determination of cariogen bacteria and salivary parameters. These tests are available since the begining of 1970s years. Using these products allows semiquantitative evaluation of mutans streptococci in saliva or plaque and lactobacilli in saliva (Larmas, 1975; Jensen & Bratthall, 1989).

Earlier test systems (Dentocult SM, Dentocult LB from Orion Diagnostica, Cariescreen SM from APO Diagnostics, Caries Check SM and Caries Check LB from Hain Diagnostika) needed relatively complicated laboratory working procedures. The newer type of Dentocult tests allows simpler technical work but they work on the same basis.

3.2.1.1 Estimation of mutans streptococci

The basis of the determination of streptococcus mutans is represented by a basic method of Dentocult SM test could be used for estimation of mutans streptococci. Originally it has been developed by Jensen & Bratthall (1989), but this Dentocult SM (Strip Mutans) is a newer development of the spatula method of Köhler & Bratthall (1979). The test is based on those facts that adhesing of mutans streptococci can be experienced not only to tooth surface but to wooden or plastic spatulas and removable devices also and on the ability of mutans streptococci to grow on hard surfaces and use of a selective broth (high sucrose concentration in combination with bacitracin). The test result shows the risk of caries depending on the level of mutans streptococci CFU (Colony Forming Units/ml) in saliva or in dental plaque, but the result has to be interpreted in relation to the number of the teeth in the mouth (Zickert et al., 1982). An other type of the available simple and accurate chairside test is „Saliva – Check mutans" from the GC, which detects the patients level of streptococcus mutans in 15 minutes only. For this test there is no need for incubator (in contrast with the previously mentioned product) or any other devices. High accuracy is possible as the test strip contains 2 monoclonal antibodies that selectively detect only the streptococcus mutans species, meaning no other bacteria modify the results.

3.2.1.2 Estimation of lactobacilli

The other organisms that can be associated with caries are lactobacilli. Althoug probably they don't play a primary role in the etiology of caries, lactobacilli can be important from the viewpoint of caries activity (Socransky, 1968). Based on different studies the presence of lactobacilli reflects only high consumption of carbohydrates and therefore it is an indirect test for caries (Klock & Krasse, 1979; Crossner, 1981). On the other hand the test provides information about the activity of existing carious lesions (high levels of lactobacilli show an incresed carious activity which can lead to early treatment of the lesions).

For the estimation of lactobacilli can be used a method of dip slide test (Larmas, 1975). The applied selective lactobacillus agar which supports the grows of the acid forming and acid resistant lactobacilli (mainly Lactobacillus casei). The dip slide has to be placed into the transport tube and incubated for four days at 37 °C (99 °F). Estimation of lactobacilli, similarly to mutans streptococci, can be performed by comparing the result to the chart. For the evaluation the number of the colonies means the relevant information. Because of different incubation times for the various test vials and the short shelf life of the mutans streptococci tests, further efforts have been made for optimize the tests in accordance with the practical viewpoints.

3.2.1.3 CRT bacteria test for combined determination of cariogenic bacteria

The prognosis for caries risk is more certain in those case when mutans streptococci and lactobacillus tests are combined (Stecksen-Blicks, 1985). CRT Bacteria (Vivadent, Shaan, Lichtenstein) (Figure 8.) is a test which is available for the evaluation of the level both important oral microorganisms by means of selective agars as previously described.

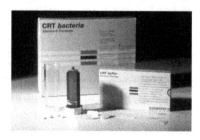

Fig. 8. CRT Bacteria test.

This test give a possibility for the determining mutans streptococci and lactobacilli at the same time, during the evaluation of caries risk.

Performing the clinical procedures, after two days incubation at 37 °C (99 °F) can be detected and evaluated for both mutans streptococci and lactobacilli. Leaving CRT bacteria in the incubator for more than 48 hours for any reason, it will not cause any change in bacterial count. The test sample can be stored in the refrigerator for up to two weeks without any changes.

Evaluation of the CRT bacteria test (with the model chart): higher values than 10^5 CFU/mL of mutans streptococci in saliva indicate a high risk (Krasse, 1988; Anderson et al., 1993). CRT bacteria test can be applied to check the effectiveness of different antimicrobial treatment of the risk patients. The modification of the above presented procedure gives a possibility for the determination of mutans streptococci not only in saliva but in dental plaque also, but applying this saliva based method, the examination of incubated plaque samples provides only a semiquantitative evaluation of the microorganisms (Kneist et al., 1998). This measure is indicated to monitor the the edges around brackets in orthodontic patients.

The tests are contraindicated after treatment with previous antibiotic treatment (within the previous two weeks) or after the use of antibacterial rinsing solution (the waiting time at least 12 hours).

All tests are very easy to use, can be applied to demonstrate the proper oral hygiene and to check the effects of motivation, generally less expensive than conventional microbiological methods (Newbrun et al., 1984) and do not need specially trained personnel. These are important diagnostic tools for dentists who strive to maintain oral health of their patients.

Presently the trends towards using simple, quick tests which can demonstrate the results clearly (without any other special equipments like e.g. incubator) for the patients in a short time. These tests are based on various methods: e.g. monoclonal antibodies are employed in Saliva Check Mutans from GC, Clinpo ™ Cario L-Pop ™ from 3M need local measurement of acid production for assessment. This last test was used in a 12 month follow up cohort study to evaluate the association between having a high score on this test and caries occurance in young patients undergoing orthodontic treatment (Chaussain et al., 2010). More studies are needed for the evaluation because of basic method of these tests not yet fully matured in terms of their sensitivity and handling properties.

3.2.2 Assessment of salivary factors

Salivary factors are in closed connection with caries risk. Determination of salivary enzymes and ions is difficult in the everyday practice, but measurement of salivary flow rate (the volume of saliva during a given period of time) or salivary buffer capacity can be performed relatively easily.

3.2.2.1 Salivary flow rate

It is wellknown for a long time that in patients with xerostomia the caries rate is increased. So the measurement of this factor must be of interest to evaluate the potentially high risk groups of orthodontic patients. The flow rate can be established easily without any special equipments. The saliva has to be collected in calibrated tube (tube for the lactobacillus test can be used to measure the salivary flow rate as well) (Figure 9.). Secretion rate should be determined for resting saliva and paraffin stimulated saliva. The values for the determination are shown in the Table 1.

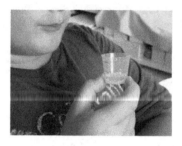

Fig. 9. Collecting saliva in a calibrated container.

For determining the risk of caries the dentist should measure the salivary secretation rate.

For the adults stimulated salivary flow rate is less than 0.7 ml/min is considered low, while higher than 1.0 mL/min is considered normal. In case of women the salivary flow rate is generally slightly lower than in men (similarly to the children when compared with the adolescents).

Secretion rate (ml/min)	Very low	Low	Normal
Resting saliva	< 0.1	0.1 - 0.25	0.25-0.35 (mean 0.30)
Stimulated saliva	< 0.7	0.7 - 1	1 – 3 (mean 2)

Table 1. Classification of salivary secretion rate for resting and paraffin-stimulated whole saliva (Axelsson, 2000).

The results could be affected by different drug intake (e.g. antihistamines, neuroleptic or antihypertensive agents).

3.2.2.2 Buffer capacity

Buffering capacity of saliva ensures the pH level and ability for remineralization. The threshold is *under* 4 when the process of caries can become faster. For the evaluation can be easily used e.g. Dentobuff strip test also from the Vivadent. A disposable syringe is used to place a single drop paraffin stimulated saliva on a test strip. After about five minutes the color change on the pH indicator strip is compared with the color chart provided. Similar possibility for measuring buffering capacity is Saliva Check Buffer from the GC.

Although it can be important information, the determination of buffer capacity, similarly to the salivary flow rate, has only subordinate role in the reliable identification of patients at high caries risk. The buffer capacity test has greater value in those patients who have exposed root surfaces because exposed dentin is more sensitive to acid than the enamel (Heintze et al, 1999).

3.3 Determination and assessment of the risk of periodontal diseases

Development and progression of periodontitis basically depends on the interaction of periodontopathogenic bacteria and the host's immune defense system. Science has long sought a diagnostic procedure to predict the risk of periodontitis with determination of the attack and defense mechanisms. For the daily practice, clinical parameters are sufficient to identify patients with potential disease activity. Periodontal diseases are in tight connection with systemic diseases (eg. cardiovascular diseases, diabetes etc.), and there is an evidence that periodontitis associated bacteria or their tissue derived inflammatory mediators are transmitted eg. during pregnancy from mother to child (Genco, 1996; Herzberg & Meyer, 1996; Slavkin, 1997). There are some chairside test which can measure different parameteres associated with periodontitis development. However, it is not clear how these tests could be clinically significant. According to several recently published reviews, none of the available tests is capable identify with at least 80% accuracy those individuals who are at risk for periodontitis (Lang & Bragger, 1991; Jeffcoat et al., 1997). Therefore, clinical evaluation seems to be more useful to carry out periodontal diagnosis and assessment the risk. The dentist has to determine the following points (Heintze et al, 1999):

1. Does gingival bleeding appear on probing?
2. Do periodontal pockets exist and how deep are they?
3. Are alterations of periodontal bone apparent on radiographs (for this periapical, bitewing and panoramic pictures are needed)

3.3.1 Clinical measurements

Greater plaque accumulation, tendency for bleeding and increased pocket depth have been observed more frequently in orthodontic patients. Therefore, to examine these factors are necessary to determine and monitor a risk of periodontal disease concerning orthodontic treatment.

3.3.1.1 Gingival Bleeding Index

Gingival Bleeding Index published by Ainamo & Bay (1975) is very simply to use in orthodontic patients. The sulcus is probed carefully on the buccal and lingual surfaces with periodontal probe. It is useful to develop a specific system e.g. to proceed by quadrants. Probing begins on the buccal surface, proceeding from the distal to mesial surfaces, then on the lingual surface from the distal to mesial. Thus each tooth has four points of measurement: buccal, lingual, mesioproximal and distoproximal.

In patient with fixed appliance performing the probing can be more difficult due to bands and other attachments limiting access to the gingival margin (Figure 10.). Still, it is necessary to probe the gingival margin along its entire length to get valuable data and to perform adequate preventive interventions.

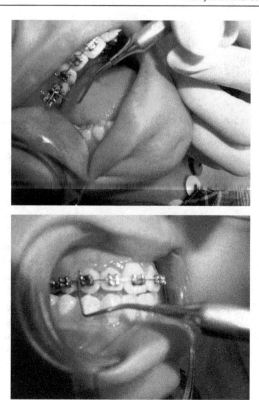

Fig. 10. Performing clinical measurements for the evaluation of periodontal conditions with a periodontal probe in orthodontic patients.

Although periodontal parameters are very important for the determination of the risk or the exist of periodontal diseases due to orthodontic treatment, sometimes it is difficult to perform because of different parts of the appliance.

3.3.1.2 Loss of attachment

The gingival sulcus is probed gently with a special periodontal probe. The depth of the gingival sulcus is considered maximally 0.5 mm deep in case of sound gingiva. In some orthodontic cases (mainly in adult patients) the measuring loss of attachment and its documentation are important, but measurement of attachment loss does not correlate with inflammatory activity of a pocket (Lang & Bragger, 1991).

3.3.2 RT-PCR (Reverse Transcription –Polymerase Chain Reaction)

One of the newest method is the RT-PCR. This is the most sensitive technique for mRNA detection and quantification currently available. It is a fully automated process and exact quantification of anaerob periodontopathogenic bacteria from a small sample of dental plaque. The advantages of this method are high specificity, high sensitivity and objectivity (Dharmaraj, 2011).

In addition to clinical and radiographic parameters and additional data provide information about the groups at higher risk for periodontitis (Fox, 1992). Patients are in higher risk in the following cases:

1. Heavy mokers
2. Diabetics
3. Patients with osteoporosis
4. Persons with inproper oral hygiene
5. Patients with previous periodontal disease
6. Elderly patients

The clinicians must identify susceptible patients and develop strategies to prevent loss of attachment and/or gingival recession. Each patient must be assessed individually for periodontal factors which mean for the patients high risk of developing periodontal disease during orthodontic treatment (Vanarsdall, 2000).

4. Possibilities to avoid or reduce the risk of caries and periodontal diseases concerning orthodontic treatment

Concerning the orthodontic treatment removable appliances do not cause significant plaque accumulation, while patients with fixed orthodontic appliances have a higher risk for increased plaque formation and with its harmful consequences for demineralization of the teeth and periodontal problems. Most of the lesions occure during fixed orthodontic treatment and appear mainly to be surface demineralization rather than a subsurface lesion. De-and remineralization processes are performed continuously. Sometimes the amount of remineralization can not totally overcome the amount of demineralization (Wilmot, 2008).

Longitudinal studies have shown the beneficial effects of recommendation to perform preventive measures during orthodontic treatment mainly in case of fixed appliances. Applying the possibilities, in these patients there was no clinically significant damage on either hard tissues of the teeth or periodontium (Boyd et al., 1989; Zachrisson & Zachrisson, 1971). Beside of the orthodontists, the general dentists and oral hygienists have a significant role in maintaining proper and effective oral hygiene of the patients undergoing orthodontic treatment with fixed appliances.

4.1 Patients with removable appliances

Although removable orthodontic appliances do not increases alone the absolute level of pathogenic microorganisms, but frequently provide more retention places for bacterial deposits (Figure 11.). In these cases the aim of oral hygienic procedures is the elimination of plaque from the appliance to prevent reinfection of the cleaned teeth. It is very difficult to keep the removable appliance totally free of plaque. Different cleaning methods are recommended mainly for home care. The orthodontist can suggest to clean with toothbrush and toothpaste (or soap) under running water or to clean the appliance in water bath containig a cleanser tablet. Both of them show some disadvantages: the combination of toothbrush-toothpaste cleaning is effective only on the easily accessible surfaces (Diedrich,

1989), while the use of self acting cleansing tablet allows just 2-3% of total deposits remaining on the appliances (Rabe et al., 1986). The antibacterial effectiveness of these tablet cleansers is doubtful and they can lead to obvious corrosion of the metal solder connections (Rabe et al.,1986). One more possibility for cleaning the removable appliances can be an ultrasonic bath, which is an expensive method and is not affordable for all patients wearing removable orthodontic appliances.

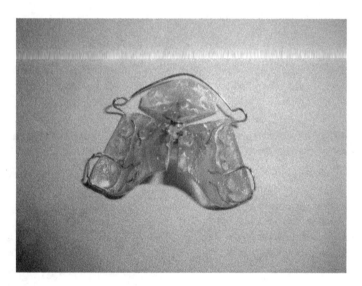

Fig. 11. Removable appliance with many retention sites and bacterial deposits.

In case of removable appliance it is necessary to clean the appliance to prevent reinfection of the cleaned teeth.

In the literature different materials are mentioned for reducing the level of pathogenic bacteria in the mouth. E.g. application of SRD (Slow Release Dosage) of chlorhexidine on the tooth surface showed a plaque reducing effect (Friedman et al., 1985), but other material with the same ingredient (e.g. Cervitec varnish) can be used effectively. Cervitec can successfully reduce cariogenic bacteria like mutans streptococci on different tooth surfaces, and promote the plaque reducing effect in the mouth (Huizinga et al., 1990; Petersson et al., 1991; Twetman & Petersson, 1997; Madléna et al., 2000). Slow release fluoride devices also can be used in case of high risk patients with removable appliances, although these products are preferred for patients treated with fixed appliances. Using slow fluoride release containing polymethyl metacrylate (Orthocryl Plus) ensures continuous low concentration of fluoride in saliva for more months which provides an optimal circumstance for the remineralization of initial carious lesions (Miethke & Newesely, 1988; Alacam et al., 1996). In case of patients using removable appliance to perform all dental and gingival treatment should be offered before the begining of the treatment.

4.2 Patients with fixed appliances

For the proper effects preventive actions and interventions should begin as early as possible, long before the active orthodontic therapy both in removable and fixed applience cases, but especially important for patients with fixed appliances.

There are three main categories should be considered concerning the preventive program for orthodontic patients: preventive actions and interventions *before, during and after* the active orthodontic treatment (Table 2.).

Before	During	After
Motivation of the patients and oral hygienic training		
Control of oral hygiene		
Dietary counselling		
Professional tooth cleaning (repeatedly if it seems to be necessary)		
	Special oral hygienic instructions concerning the fixed orthodontic appliance	
	Use of fluorides	
	Chemical plaque control	Chemical plaque control in case of fixed retainer
		Remineralization

Table 2. Preventive viewpoints before, during and after the active orthodontic treatment with fixed orthodontic appliance (Lundström et al., 1980; Hotz, 1982).

In all patients but especially in case of fixed appliance it is very important that all general dental and periodontal treatment should be completed *before* orthodontic treatment. It is compulsory to consult with the general dentist or any specialist to gain a statement that the patient is ready for orthodontic treatment. To prepare a written inform consent including the necessity of improved oral hygiene is also necessary before begining of the treatment. The oral condition has also to be recorded on the patient's chart and demonstrated with clinical photos.

Concerning the treatment, bonding of molars is better and ensures better possibilities to remove the plaque than banding, especially in adults. For the same reason it is suggested to use single arch wires, if the case allows and to remove excess composite around brackets (mainly from the gingival third). Theoretically use of fluoride containing orthodontic adhesives are preferable during orthodontic treatment and in case of fixed retainer. In vitro studies glass ionomer cements have demonstrated a more sustained fluoride release and evidence that these cements may reduce decalcification (Vorhies et al., 1998; Chung et al., 1999; Millett et al., 1999). At the same time, according to a systematic review, glass ionomer cement could be more effective than composite resin in preventing white spot formation, but still the scientific evidence is weak. The authors conclude that fluoride releasing bonding material for bonding brackets showed almost no demineralization-inhibiting effect (Derks et al., 2004).

Because of the limitation of successful bonding with glass ionomer adhesives, further investigations are needed for the recommendations on the usage of fluoride containing adhesives during fixed orthodontic treatment (Rogers et al., 2010). Uysal et al. (2011) conclude that using antibacterial monomer containing adhesive for bonding orthodontic brackets successfully inhibited caries incidence in vivo, the cariostatic effect was localized around the brackets and proved to be significant after 30 days.

Lingual appliances can cause extra difficulties in performing proper oral hygiene. The longer the treatment time with fixed appliance, the more time needed to maintain oral health in such a non-ideal circumstance. It is preferable to minimize the length of treatment with either conventionally or lingually placed fixed orthodontic appliance (e.g. by early corrections of skeletal and alignment problems in the mixed dentition with removable appliances). In addition a light cure sealant containing fluoride should also be advisable to be applied on the entire free surface, which can also be reapplied during the treatment (Frazier et al., 1996). Fluoride containing elastomeric chains also may reduce the degree of decalcification (Banks et al., 2000).

4.2.1 Motivation of the patients and oral hygienic training; control of oral hyiene

Before the orthodontic treatment it is very important to inform the patients about the importance of the improved oral hygiene concerning orthodontic treatment with fixed appliance and to explain the causes of caries and periodontal disease. The dentist can use any gingival indices and disclosure of the plaque for the patient to be motivated. The patients need proper information about the preventive possibilities concerning fixed orthodontic appliance after its application. It could be very useful to check the oral hygiene throught the complete orthodontic therapy. Beside of the use of fluoride containing toothpaste and brushing with conventional brushes also during the treatment at least twice a day, additional methods could be suggested helping to improve oral hygiene. Recording and documentation of the improvement in oral hygiene in the patient's chart is also necessary. Although motivation and oral hygiene training represent the most important points before the orthodontic treatment, it can be repeated as frequently as it is needed not only before but during the active orthodontic treatment as well. *After finishing the orthodontic treatment* the orthodontist also has to advice the patients to maintain proper oral hygienic habits.

4.2.2 Oral hygienic training methods

It is a possibility and a responsibility of the orthodontists to involve their patients in a systemic program for the prevention of caries and periodontal diseases focusing on mechanical removal of plaque and elimination of pathogen microorganisms. Because of tooth cleaning is much more difficult in patients undergoing orthodontic therapy with fixed appliance, patients and orthodontists/dentists or specially trained personnel require much efforts and time to show the possibilities of proper oral hygiene. Ask the patients to demonstrate the efficiency of brushing at each regular visit until they have mastered the technique.

The patients can use both hand or electric tooth brushes with short head, soft and rounded bristle end, but they can apply special orthodontic brushes (eg. when middle row of bristles is shorter than the outer row) and have to ask other special equipments also (eg. floss, interdental brushes, etc.) (Figure 12.). The patients may be instructed in the modified Bass technique. It is also important to let the toothbrush air-dried for 24 hours between uses. Tooth cleaning requires at least 10 minutes for patients. Approximal surfaces could be cleaned properly with dental floss. Interdental brushes and Superfloss must be used for the proper oral hygiene not only on the approximal surfaces but the tooth surfaces around the bracket and band margins as well (Heintze et al., 1999; Boyd, 2001).

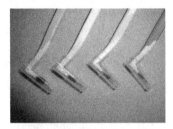

Fig. 12. Special brushes for orthodontic patients.

During the orthodontic treatment with fixed appliance it is necessary to suggest special equipments for the proper oral hygiene and to check the effectiveness of them.

4.2.3 Control of oral hygiene

During the active treatment patients should evaluate their teeth (and appliances) and determine these are whether clean or not. Regular recall examinations are necessary but the intervals between the recall examinations depend on the initial conditions. At the recall examinations during both the active treatment phase and the retention period regularly should perform the determination of caries risk (mutans streptococci and lactobacilli counts) and the evaluation of the condition of gingiva.

During the retention phase, removable retainers mean lower risk because these appliances allow an easier tooth cleaning procedure. The attached fixed retainers represent plaque retentive sites in the mouth, although these appliances are believed not to lead to initial carious lesions or periodontal problems if properly fabricated (Artun, 1984; Gorelick et al., 1982). Further advantage of removable devices is that they could be used as carriers of medicaments to provide more intensive prophylaxis.

4.2.4 Dietary counselling

Sugar is not a single causative factor of dental caries but it can appear as an important external modifying risk factor in this process. Due to this reason the dental personnel have to ask the patients about their nutritional habits, optimally using a questionnaire. It is very important to know the average frequency of intake of any types of the cariogenic foods (Axelsson, 1999).

The dietary control is in close connection with microbiologic evaluations. As high salivary levels of lactobacilli indicate a high sugar intake and a low pH in the oral cavity, the lactobacillus test is useful for the objective supplement to the dietary questionnaire (Axelsson, 1999). Sugar intake can be assessed eg. from a 24 hour recall questionnaire. For caries prevention and control the following dietary recommendations should be performed for the patients according to Axelsson (1999):

1. The first meal of the day (breakfast), should be a balanced composition of dairy products, grains and fruit eg. yogurt and muesli, fresh fruit and vegetables. It is not the same as the commercial continental breakfast containing mainly fat, sugar and water which causes rapid swings in blood sugar levels stimulating a high frequency of sugar intake all day.
2. The total number of meals, including all, should be limited to about four.
3. Sticky, sugar containing products should be eliminated. Sugarless sweets containing sugar substitutes (xylitol, sorbitol, aspartam etc.) should be used.
4. In each meal, fiber rich products that stimulate chewing and salivary flow should be included.
5. Selected individuals with extremely high risk of development of caries should clean all surfaces just before each meal, to limit the drop in pH during and immediately after the meal.

4.2.5 Professional tooth cleaning

Professional tooth cleaning represents a basic method and means professional removal of all deposits from the teeth by dentist, dental hygienist or specially trained nurses. For the proximal surfaces dental floss must be used (and fissures must be sealed if indicated). Calculus (mineralized plaque) can be removed with manual or ultrasonic scalers, after it the teeth should be polished. A complete professional tooth cleaning should be performed before the active orthodontic treatment and at the appointments of control examinations.

4.2.6 Use of fluorides

A correlation between reduced caries prevalence and natural fluoride content of drinking water was published firstly by Dean (1938). Saliva usually contains a low amount of fluoride (Twetman et al., 1999). The importance of fluoridation is basic to maintain the health of teeth, particularly in the prevention of caries and remineralization of incipient carious lesions. A report published by the WHO (1994) and a review article by Rolla et al. (1991) state that the use of fluoridated tooth paste had led to a significant decrease in the incidence of caries in the industrialized countries. The ability of fluoride to retard or prevent the development of dental caries appears to involve several mechanisms including a reduction in the acid solubility of enamel, promotion of enamel remineralization, inhibition of glucose uptake and utilization by acidogenic bacteria. Demineralization refers to the loss of minerals (mainly calcium and phosphate ions) from the tooth structure due to the acidic and cariogenic challenge. Fluoride can help to prevent the mineral loss. When the pH drops below approximately 5.5, calcium ions are dissolved from the enamel and bond with fluoride ions forming a calcium fluoride (CaF_2) layer (Rolla & Saxegaard, 1990). CaF_2 is insoluble in the saliva and remains on the teeth for months (Dijkman et al., 1983). The CaF_2 layer functions as a pH controlled fluoride reservoir and is the most important supplier of free fluoride ions during the cariogen challenge (Fischer et al., 1995). Fluoride uptake and release of the enamel are strongly dependent on the duration of contact with the fluoridated agent (Ten Cate & Arends, 1980; Chen et al., 1985). With an appropriate fluoride formulation, incipient lesions could be reduced in size or even be repaired (Tranaeus et al., 2001).

Research suggests that topical fluorides might also decrease decalcification during orthodontic treatment (Geiger et al., 1988; Shannon & West, 1979; Benson et al., 2004; Derks et al., 2004; Chadwick et al., 2005; Sudjalim et al, 2006). Daily use of fluoride toothpaste, in combination with specific oral hygienic instructions, is recommended as the basis of caries and periodontal prophylaxis programme. Although fluoride concentration in different products may vary, below 0.1% in a dentifrice is not recommended for orthodontic patients (Ogaard et al., 2004). There are a number of locally applicable agents to improve maintain proper oral hygiene. The most important aim with the fluoridated dental care products first of all to strengthen of enamel against to caries, enhance the remineralization, protection against demineralization and improve or ensure gingival health. Beside of the toothpaste, fluoridated agents are included in different forms of gels, mouthrinses, varnishes and other products.

Topical fluoride may be applied by professional personnel in dental office or by patients at home. Using other local fluoridaton's method, a balance should be maintain between the prevention of dental caries and minimising the risk of dental mottling (Oulis et al., 2009). Generally, dentifrice alone is ineffective in preventing development of lesions (O'Reilly & Featherstone, 1987).

4.2.6.1 Fluoride rinses

Relevant studies have shown that daily use of fluoride rinse during the orthodontic treatment can reduce the incidence of initial carious lesions. At the same time, relatively few of orthodontic patients rinsed daily with fluoride containing mouthrinses (Geiger et al., 1988).

It has been published that caries reduction with different mouthrinses was estimated 25-30 % (Geiger et al., 1988; Newbrun, 1992). Rinses generally contain 0.025 to 0.05 % sodium fluoride, 0.025 % amine fluoride, 0.01 % zinc fluoride or 0.025 % APF (Acidulated Phosphate Fluoride), but more highly concentrated solutions are recommended for patients with increased risk (Zachrisson, 1975). Patients in high caries risk such as orthodontic patients should use a daily rinse of eg. 0.05% sodium fluoride at home (Petersson, 1993). Fluoride containing mouthrinse can be used at a time that is different to any tooth brushing for an additive effect to fluoride toothpaste (Oulis et al., 2009) or after the toothbrushing to complete the fluoride intake.

4.2.6.2 Fluoride gels

Fluoride containing gels can be used on patients yearly or half-yearly in dental office or can be used regularly by the patient, at home. The application of fluoride gels can reduce the occurance of caries by 21-30 % (Marinho et al., 2002; Marthaler, 1988).

4.2.6.3 Fluor protector gel

The Fluor Protector Gel (Vivadent, Shaan, Liechtenstein) contains calcium (Ca), phosphate and 1450 ppm fluoride (F) forming a CaF_2 layer and a direct incorporation of Ca, fluoride and phosphate ions into the tooth enamel. CaF_2 preferably deposits on demineralized surfaces and this layer is additionally stabilised by phosphate ions (Rolla and Saxegaard, 1990), which are also contained in Fluor Protector Gel. If the pH falls into the acidic range, the calcium fluoride layer releases Ca and phosphate ions which are released into the saliva and form a depot. It will work against demineralization or can contribute to the formation of fluoro-apatite or fluoro-hydroxyl-apatite. This replacement of hydroxy ion by a fluoride ion in the hydroxy apatite ensures the tooth enamel with higher resistance to pH drops (Fischer et al., 1995).

The Fluor Protector Gel can either used by the dentist in the dental surgery or by the patients at home, in different ways. It can be used in place of toothpaste to brush the teeth, or in the evening, after cleaning the teeth with toothpaste, when Fluor Protector Gel can be additionally applied with the toothbrush. It is suggested for cleaning interdental spaces of natural dentition or fixed dental restorations etc.. It also can be used with a tray filled with gel inserting it once or twice daily, and leaving it in place for 10 minutes every occasion.

It is especially recommended in high risk patients undergoing orthodontic treatment with fixed appliances.

4.2.6.4 Stannous fluoride gel

Since the late 1970s, 0.4% stannous fluoride (SnF_2) gels have been widely used as therapeutic agents for number of common oral diseases and conditions, and promoted as the preferred preventive and treatment products (Hastreiter, 1989; Paraskevas & van der Weiden, 2006). It contains more than 90% available stannous ion (Sn^{2+}) which is useful againts either plaque accumulation or gingivitis.

4.2.6.5 Halitosis tooth and tongue gel, Amine fluoride gel (see below)

4.2.6.6 Amine fluoride/ amine and stannous fluoride containing products

The use of amine fluorides in dentistry was recommended firstly by Mühlemann et al. (1957). The beneficial effects of them are well known as protective agents against mainly caries and dental plaque accumulation (Schmid, 1983; Öhrn & Sanz, 2009). These products were used in the form of dentifrices, gels and fluids in various caries preventive programs and suggested as alternatives or adjunctives for systemic fluoridation. Clinical studies with amine fluorides can be divided into trials with dentifrice only, with gel only or combined use of these products similarly to the use of mouthrinse and/or toothpaste. Fluoride containing gels are recommended annually or semiannually in the dental office. By the patients' home use, it is suggested to brush once a week, after a regular toothbrusing. Gels contain high concentration of different types of fluorides. Gels containing amine fluoride (in 12 500 ppm concentration) (Elmex gel, Gaba Int. Ltd., Switzerland) are used mostly in Europe. The active ingredients of the clinically tested relatively new product (Halitosis tooth and tongue gel) (Gaba Int. Ltd., Switzerland) (Figure 13.) are amine fluoride/ stannous fluoride and zinc lactate). This gel protects against caries, cleans the teeth and tongue (by helping a special tongue cleaner) and even neutralizes odour-active compounds in the oral cavity. It is offered for adults and childrens above the age of 12 years. It is also very useful for orthodontic patients with fixed orthodontic appliances because of these appliances can cause oral malodour (Babacan et al., 2011). This product is available in the form as mouthrinse with 250 ppm fluoride content.

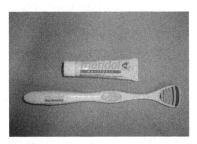

Fig. 13. Halitosis tooth and tongue gel and a tongue scraper.

This product is very useful for the patients undergoing orthodontic treatment.

Clinical trials with amine fluoride toothpaste, performed between 1968 and 1995 with a duration of 2.5-7 years, has reported reduction in mean DMFT/DMFS of between 7.1 and 35 % (Marthaler, 1968; 1974; Patz & Naujoks, 1970; Ringelberg et al., 1979; Cahen et al., 1982; Leous et al.,1995). Studies with amine fluoride gel between 1970 and 1989 with a duration of 1.5-7 years reported caries reductions of 31 - 53 % (Marthaler et al., 1970; Shern et al., 1976; Franke et al., 1977; Obersztyn & Kolwinski, 1984; Szőke & Kozma, 1989). In a 7-year clinical study using a combination of amine fluoride products a 43% reduction in DMFS mean values was found (Künzel et al., 1977). Madléna et al. (2002) published significant reduction in DMFS value (38 % including white spot lesions) and 34 % (not including white spot lesions) and a significant reduction in Plaque Index values with the combined use of amine fluoride containing toothpaste and gel in a high risk groups of adolescents. Márton et al. (2008) published beneficial effects of amine fluoride products.

The effects of Sn_2F or AmF/Sn_2F containing products on plaque accumulation were examined by many investigators (Øgaard et al., 1980; Bánóczy et al., 1989; Zimmermann et al., 1993; Mengel et al., 1996; Madléna et al., 2004; Gerardu et al., 2007). Madléna et al. (2009) proved the beneficial effects of amine fluoride /stannous fluoride containing products on periodontal parameters in patients treated with fixed orthodontic appliances. However, during a short term (four week-) examination period, there was no found significant difference between the groups using amine fluoride containing toothpaste only and the other group with combined use of toothpaste and mouthrinse containing the same ingredient. Although, at the same time numbers of streptococcus mutans and lactobacilli were reduced and level of periopathogen microorganisms also showed a very impressive decrease after even a four weeks use (Madléna et al., 2009; Nagy et al, 2010).

4.2.6.7 Fluoride varnishes

The development of fluoride varnishes started after the study of Mellberg et al. (1966). These authors found that considerable amounts of fluoride were released from enamel within the first 24 hours following the topical application of acidulated fluoride phosphate preparations. APF (Acidulated Phosphate Fluoride) increases the uptake of fluoride into the enamel because of its low pH. It is used mostly in the US. Schmid (1964) presented a topical fluoride method using a varnish with a high fluoride concentration. It was the Duraphat (Colgate Oral Pharmaceutical Inc., Canton, USA) which had the ability to adhere to tooth surfaces in the presence of saliva. Duraphat varnish consists of a natural resin (colophonium base with 5 % sodium fluoride (2.23 % F-) dissolved in ethanol. It hardens the enamel in contact with saliva producing a temporary cover over the enamel. The patient is instructed to refrain from brushing for four hours after application (Retief et al, 1985; Staley 2008). The varnish also leaves calcium fluoride on the surface of the enamel in a CaF_2-like material that is less soluble and most likely leaches away from the surface through the pellicle (Dijkman & Arends, 1988). The other similar varnish system (Fluor protector) (Vivadent, Shaan, Liechtenstein) was introduced by Arends and Schuthof in 1975. Fluor protector contains 0.1 % F- as difluorosilane dissolved in ethyl acetate and isoalylpropionate solution which has acidic properties. It is advisable that the patients avoid rinsing after application. Eating or brushing the teeth should also be avoided at least 45 minutes after the treatment. The differences can be found between the two varnishes are important in solvent, fluoride concentration, consistency, hardening time, colour, scent and taste. The varnishes coat the tooth surfaces as a thin layer that hardens a few minutes after application. The cost benefit ratio of fluoride varnishes is better then that of gels, and these products ensure the elimination the problem of compliance, as they are applied professionally (two to four times per year).

Beside of the above mentioned two types of fluoride varnish there are some other products. Duraflor (DenTrek, registered trademark of OMNI™ Preventive Care) is a 5 % NaF varnish containing xylitol and a bubble gum flavouring. Cavity shield contains 5% NaF in a neutral resin. The fluoride content is reported more uniform than that of Duraphat (Shen & Autio-Gold, 2002). The unit dose can be mixed easily and applied to teeth (Chu & Lo, 2006). Bifluorid 12 (Oceanwealth Horizon , (Voco), Düsseldorf, Germany) contains both NaF (2.7% F) and CaF_2 (2.9 % F). This combination of fluoride allows more fluoride deposit on the surface of demineralized enamel than NaF varnish alone (Attin et al., 1995).

Clinical studies showed beneficial effects of fluoride varnishes on caries reduction in both permanent and deciduous dentitions (Marinho, 2004). In the permanent dentition it was ranged from 20-70% compared to untreated controls (Petersson, 1975; de Bruyn & Arends, 1987), although it is very important to consider that clinical results are strongly influenced by different factors (e.g. caries prevalence, frequency of application of the varnish, caries risk etc.). Fluoride varnishes should be considered for use as a preventive adjunctive method to reduce demineralization adjacent to orthodontic brackets, especially in patients exhibiting pure compliance in oral hygiene and home fluoride use (Todd et al., 1999).

Advantages of fluoride varnishes are multiple: prolonged contact time acting as a slow release reservoir; these could be applied simply, quickly, easily; there is no need for widespread professional prophylaxis before the application of varnish because this procedure does not mean any additional effect, varnishes are safe, for even very young children. (Chu & Lo, 2006). Both parents and dentists prefer fluoride varnishes to fluoride gels (Warren et al., 2000). One disadvantage of Duraphat is its poor esthetic effect (a yellow film of varnish remains on the teeth for several hours after application) (Warren et al., 2000).

In a conclusion: there is moderate information is available on remineralization effectiveness of fluoride varnishes, but based on some investigations these could be offered for potential remineralization of the enamel (Castellano & Donly, 2004; Ogaard et al., 1984, 1996).

4.2.6.8 Slow release fluoride devices

Considering that intraoral levels of fluoride play a key role in the dynamics of dental caries, it has been suggested that the use of controlled and sustained delivery systems can be considered as a means of controlling dental caries incidence in high risk individuals (Mirth, 1980).

In a review of Pessan et al. (2008) there are three types of devices: Copolymer membrane device, Glass device, Hydroxyapatite Eudragit RS100 diffusion controlled F system. The third one is the newest type of slow release device, which consists of a mixture of hydroxyapatite, NaF and Eudragit RS100; it contains 18 mg NaF and intended to release 0.15 mg F/day. It was demonstrated that the use of this device is able to significantly increase salivary and urinary F concentration for at least 1 month (Altinova et al., 2005). These devices are effective in raising intraoral F concentrations at levels able to reduce enamel solubility, resulting in caries protective effect. The use of slow relesase devices have been shown to have a very favourable benefit regarding cost-effecitiveness ratios (Toumba, 1996). Slow release devices can show a high anticaries effect for patients in high caries risk (Featherstone, 2006). Beside of this, such a device would overcome compliance problems also. It may not eliminate all carious lesions, but would lead to dramatic reduction and in combination with antibacterial treatments could indeed eliminate caries in high risk individuals (Pessan et al., 2008).

4.2.7 Oral health care products for chemical plaque control

4.2.7.1 Chlorhexidine (CHX) containing products

Among chemical plaque control agents chlorhexidine digluconate has proven to be the most effective and safe. It seems to be the most important antimicrobial ingredient in dental products, which is available in forms of rinse, gel and varnish. Inspite of the side effects, experienced first of all with the mouthrinse, using of these products is considered as the best possibility to treat gingivitis.

4.2.7.1.1 Chlorhexidine mouthrinses

These types of clorhexidine containing products [(e.g. Corsodyl mouthrinses (GlaxoSmithKline, Brentford, UK)] are the most frequently used form in dentistry for patients with gingivitis and periodontitis and before or after surgical procedures. Professionally chlorhexidine solution could be used for irrigation the inflammed pockets. Anderson et al. (1997) published that use of CHX mouthrinse in addition to regular oral hygiene was effective in reducing plaque and gingivitis in adolescents undergoing orthodontic treatment. Ready to use 0.1 or 0.2 % mouthrinses are available. Löe et al. (1972) published that twice daily rinsing with an 0.2% CHX solution reduced the total bacterial count in saliva by 85-90%. In practice, it is offered for twice-daily use for a limited, 6 week term because of the side effects of this agent. These are the discoloration of the teeth, fillings and tongue, taste disturbances (hot and bitter) in the mouth. It can leave an unpleasant aftertaste and repeated use lead to an impaired sense of taste and desquamations.

Based on the available reviews, chlorhexidine rinses have not been highly effective in preventing caries or at least the clinical data are not convincing (Autio-Gold, 2008). Due to the current lack of long term clinical evidence for caries prevention and reported side effect, CHX rinses should not really be recommended for caries prevention. However, the use of gels, and varnishes should also be studied further on to have evidence-based recommendations for their clinical role in caries prevention (Autio-Gold, 2008).

4.2.7.1.2 Chlorhexidine gels

Treatment with gel seems to be more effective than treatment with mouthrinse because the gel adheres to the tooth surface for longer period. Emilson (1981) published that CHX containing gel inhibited the plaque formation on tooth surfaces, effected on Gram positive and Gram negative bacteria such as mutans streptococci. CHX containing gel (e.g. Corsodyl with 1% CHX) (GlaxoSmithKline, Brentford, UK) similarly to other gels can be applied with toothbrush or in a custom made tray. The use of tray is better because the gel can attach the tooth surface without dilution and it is not distributed on the mucosa. The CHX gel ensures significant reduction in mutans streptococci, at the same time the patient has no unpleasent sense of taste. The time tested ingredient CHX reduces the growth of harmful bacteria and yeast. So there are less plaque formed on the teeth or appliances and the inflammation of gum tissues subsides.

Because of the beneficial effects, CHX containing gel suggested to use with a special soft tray. This therapy delivered by a tray which is offered for only older children, adolescents or adults who are able to apply the gel and tray safety, otherwise the gel should be used with toothbrush or with cotton roll.

Clinical studies defined the caries inhibiting effect of CHX (Zickert et al., 1982). It was also published that the effect of CHX gel is increased with combined use of fluoride gel (Ostela & Tenovuo, 1990; Meurman, 1988). In addition to the antibacterial CHX (0.11%), Cervitec gel (Vivadent, Schaan, Liechtenstein) containing fluoride (900 ppm) which promotes remineralization and protects the teeth from caries. At the same time it is an effective antimicrobial product. Cervitec gel can be used with interdental brushes, with toothbrush, tray or it can be applied directly on the gum.

4.2.7.1.3 Chlorhexidine varnishes

During the past decade, varnishes for local delivery of antimicrobial agents have been developed and investigated in vitro and in vivo. The inhibitory effect of CHX on mutans streptococci or new carious lesions was confirmed with fixed orthodontic appliances (Lundström and Krasse, 1987; Madléna et al., 2000; Derks et al., 2004) (Figure 14.).

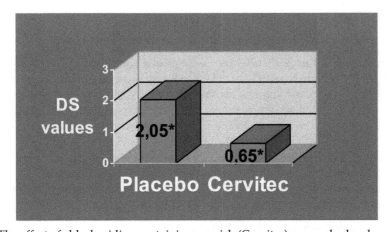

Fig. 14. The effect of chlorhexidine containing varnish (Cervitec) on newly developed carious lesions during orthodontic treatment (*p<0.05)
The number of the new carious lesions was significantly lower in the quadrants treated with Cervitec than in the quadrants treated with placebo (*p<0.05).(Madléna et al., 2000).

It has been concluded by a review that the most persistent reduction of mutans streptococci have been achived by chlorhexidine varnishes followed by gels and lastly mouthrinses (Autio-Gold, 2008). Cervitec plus is a newer, now available member of the „Cervitec family" (Vivadent, Shaan, Liechtenstein) containing chlorhexidine and thymol). Comparing three varnish systems (Chlorzoin, containing CHX 10% (Knowell Therapeutic Technologies, owned company Toronto, Canada), EC 40, containing CHX 40% (Biodent BV, Nijmegen, The Netherlands), Cervitec Plus, containing CHX 1%), a single application of a highly concentrated varnish (EC 40), is sufficient even with reduced contact time, whereas repeated applications and longer retention time required for varnishes with lower chlorhexidine concentration (Chlorzoin and Cervitec). All of the three varnish systems had a similar effect on mutans streptococci in the oral flora. However, none of these varnishes could maintain a significant suppression of mutans streptococci for a period of up to 6 months (repeated application is required for the effectiveness). Concerning the chlorhexidine containing varnishes there may be noticed some advers effects, similarly to other chlorhexidine containing products: staining of teeth and tongue, or taste disturbancies associated with accidental contact of CHX varnish with oral mucosa (Matthijs & Adriaens, 2002).

The most sensitive bacteria to chlorhexidine-thymol varnish (Cervitec plus) are Porphyromonas gingivalis and Aggregatibacter Actynomycetemcomitans. Therefore, chlorhexidine varnishes may be promising for the prevention of periodontal disease or as an adjunct to periodontal therapy (Petersson et al. 1992; Matthijs & Adriaens, 2002). Twetman and Petersson (1997) reported that a combined treatment with a chlorhexidine – thymol and a fluoride varnish resulted in a longer inhibiting effect on interdental plaque samples, than chlorhexidine-thymol varnish alone. The use of dental varnishes with antimicrobial properties might have potential benefits for patients with chronic gingival inflammation (Matthijs & Adriaens, 2002).

4.2.7.2 Other products

4.2.7.2.1 Essential oils containing products - Listerine (Johnson & Johnson, Maidenhead, UK)

Active ingredients of this oral rinse are essential oils (eucalyptol, thymol, menthol) for bactericid effect, contains methyl salicylate (against analgesia and inflammation) and alcohol (in which the active ingredients are diluted). It should be used as a rinse twice daily for 1 minute. As it does not contain any fluoride or its fluoride concentration is very low (in the newer products), has no effect on caries, but it has an antigingivitis effect According to a systematic review published by Van Leeuwen et al. (2011), in long term use, the standardized formulation of essential-oil mouthwas appeared to be a reliable alternative to chlorhexidine mouthwash with respect to parameters of gingival inflammation. Listerine toothpaste is not established as effective product against gingivitis (Boyd, 2001).

4.2.7.2.2 Triclosan-containing products - (Colgate total) (Colgate Palmolive Co. USA)

It is also an antigingivitis agent including good taste and supragingival calculus control (Volpe et al., 1996). Triclosan is available only in toothpaste (Colgate total) (Colgate Palmolive Co. USA), has an antibacterial effect and is often combined with zinc to increase the antiplaque effect. Thus, it may give potential benefits for orthodontic patients as a supplement to fluoride dentifrice during orthodontic treatment.

4.2.7.2.3 Hyaluronic acid containing products (Gengigel) (Ricefarma, Milano, Italy)

Hyaluronic acid is naturally occures as physiological constituent of connective tissue (especially in gingival mucosa). It ensures antioedematous and tissue repair functions, helps to perform an antiinflammatoric effect, so can be helpful during the orthodontic treatment with fixed appliances. The lack of hyaluronic acid is responsible for the continuation of the inflammatory condition. In these cases application of hyaluronic acid provides periodontal tissue with accelerated repair functions by preventing the deficiency of natural gingival hyaluronic acid and enhancing its effects.

The hyaluronic acid containing Gengigel can be available in forms gel, rinse and spray. Pistorius et al. (2002) published positive effects of Gengigel spray: this product ensured significant improvements in gingival parameters in case of gingivitis, after 7 days application. All Gengigel products are suggested to use in case of gingivitis, gingival bleeding, gingival pockets (also gingival recession, abrasion and other tissue trauma etc.), after the correct oral hygiene three to five times a day (after main meals) for 3-4 weeks, continuing until the symptoms have disappeared. Side effect has not been experienced with these products.

4.2.7.2.4 Antibiotics

Use of oral or systemic antibiotic therapy is indicated to eliminate specific pathogenic organisms. However, antibiotic therapy can never replace the mechanical removal of subgingival deposits and it should be only a supplemental, supportive therapy, similarly to the treatment of serious periodontal diseases, but this indication belongs to an experienced periodontist and should not be administratinly by an orthodontist.

4.3 Remineralization – Treatment of white spot lesions after removal of fixed appliance

4.3.1 Fluorides

Fluoride increses the initial rate of remineralization of early enamel lesions and slow down the progress of carious process by reacting with the minerals present in the surface of the lesion. Enamel can be remineralized with meticulous toothbrushing twice per day, with fluoridated dentifrice. Additional fluoride application can further enhance the remineralization process. This would include eg. fluoridated dentifrice with higher dose, fluoride rinses, topical fluoride gels, fluoride varnishes and professionally applied topical fluoride such as 2% sodium fluoride, 8% stannous fluoride and 1.23% acidulated phosphate fluoride (Donly & Sasa, 2008). At the same time it was published that when high doses of fluoride are used locally (mainly during the first few weeks after completed the orthodontic treatment), the arrested lesion stays the same size and frequently becomes unsightly and stained with organic debris which is esthetically not optimal on the labial surfaces (Ogaard et al., 2004; Willmot, 2008). To avoid arresting the lesion and obtunding the surface layer several authors recommended low dose fluoride applications to enhance subsurface remineralization It was published that 50 ppm fluoride mouthrinse had a higher efficiency for remineralization than control solution for regular mouthrinse containing 250 ppm (Linton, 1996; Lagerwij et al., 1997). In spite of these observations, Wilmot (2004) did not confirm the therapeutic effect of low fluoride (50 ppm) products and concluded that postorthodontic white spot lesions (WSL) reduced in size during the 6 months by approximately half of the original size, but there was no clinical advantage of using the low fluoride formulation of mouthrinse/toothpaste in this process comparing to those of using fluoride free products as a control. The mean size of the lesions reduced with time in both groups. A therapeutic effect (less than 30%) was non significant. Beside of the labial surfaces application of concentrated fluoride was suggested to prevent the progresson of the lesions. It has been also suggested that acid etching of fluoride treated lesions could facilitate remineralization of the lesions by oral fluids (Hicks et al., 1984).

4.3.2 Use of Casein Phosphopeptide-Amorphus Calcium Phosphate (CPP-ACP)

Enamel can also be remineralized with Casein Phosphopeptide-Amorphus Calcium Phosphate preparations. CPP-ACP is capable to be absorbed through the enamel surface and could affect the carious process (Reynolds, 1987) CPP-ACP system (the trade name is Recaldent™) which allows freely available calcium and phosphate ions to attach to enamel and reform into calcium phosphate crystals. The free calcium and phosphate ions released from the CPP-ACP and deposit into the enamel rods. The available types of these products: water based mousse, topical creme (these are the most frequently used forms) mouthrinses, sugarfree lozenges and chewing gum (which is not suggested for orthodontic patients).

As CPP-ACP is derived from milk casein, should not be used in patient with protein and or hydroxybenzoates allergy. Studies of the effects of CPP-ACP show a dose related increase in enamel remineralization (Sudjalim et al., 2006). These products have beneficial effects in reducing area of demineralized lesions after 4 weeks (Bröchner et al., 2011).

Using the mousse (GC Tooth Mousse) to treat post-orthodontic lesions, a thermoplastic retainer needs in which a pea sized amount of CPP-ACP mousse has been spread evenly.

After proper oral hygiene the patient places the mousse at night and wears the retainer throughout sleep. Flavouring helps to stimulate saliva flow rate which helps to rinse bacteria and food residues from the teeth and enhances the effectiveness of CPP ACP in the mouth.

The GC MI Paste Plus is a water based topical creme containing Recaldent ™ CPP-ACP and fluoride (900 ppm). It can be used on teeth at home when the patient apply the products with a tray (Figure 15.), similarly to the mousse or without a tray simply with clean finger or cotton tipped applicator and let it work for 3-5 minutes.

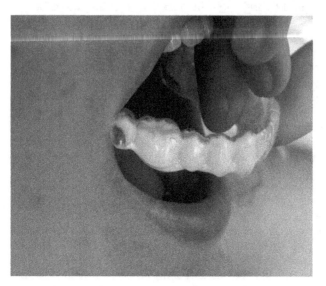

Fig. 15. Use of MI Paste Plus with a tray.

This material containing CPP ACP and fluoride can help in remineralization process e.g. after finishing the orthodontic treatment with fixed appliance

4.3.3 Microabrasion

Enamel microabrasion abrades the enamel surface, leaving a highly polished surface with Ca phosphate packed into the interprismatic enamel surface space. This highly polished enamel surface can then be bleached.

This method has been widely used for the removal of superficial non-carious enamel defects for which it can be use for example performing 18% hydrochloric acid and pumice technique (Welbury & Shaw, 1990; Rodd & Davidson, 1997). This method seems to be an effective treatment approach for cosmetic improvement of long-standing postorthodontic demineralized enamel lesions (Welbury & Carter, 1993; Croll & Bullock, 1994). Studies demonstrate that although microabrasion removes small amounts of the enamel surface, the new polished surface is less susceptible to bacterial colonization and demineralization than natural non abraded enamel (Segura et al., 1997 a,b).

Following the microabrasion technique, a 4 minute 2% sodium fluoride treatment is recommended. If the microbrasion technique could not ensure optimal esthetics and some whitened enamel is still remain, vital tooth bleaching can be considered (Donly & Sasa, 2008).

5. Conclusion

The number of orthodontic treatments among them the frequency of treatments with fixed appliances is increasing nowadays. In some cases orthodontic treatments mean caries preventive interventions when tooth movements may reliese crowding or other anomalies thus can contribute the effectiveness of proper oral hygiene. On the other hand these treatments may have causative effect on plaque induced oral diseases. For these patients effective preventive oral health care is needed and orthodontists have to be responsible for helping to keep proper oral hygiene in their patients.

The risk of caries can be determined by different tests (e.g. SM, LB chairside tests) or assessment of some salivary factors. Measurement of plaque has been found also very useful to determinate the risk of caries. The severity of periodontal diseases and the risk for these diseases can be determined by clinical measurements. Bleeding on probing remained the most certain clinical sign of periodontal inflammations. Chairside tests are available to measure different parameters associated with periodontitis, but presently there is no such a particular parameter or method predicting the possibility of periodontitis.

For prevention of caries and periodontal diseases clinicians should instruct the patients effectively to be able to perform proper oral hygiene. Regular removal of plaque and calculus at critical places can help a lot. Regular recalls, well constructed programs of regular professional oral hygiene can give great help for at-risk patients.

Beside of dietary counselling, to reduce cariogenic bacteria, use of professional and home care measures and techniques (cleaning instruments, fluoridated paste, restorative methods, application of fluoride and chlorhexidine containig materials, plaque disclosing products, special toothbrushes and other equipments etc.) could provide help.

Because of the increasing number of patients in need of orthodontic appliances, this chapter is important and useful not only for orthodontists, but general dentists or periodontists and dental students as well.

6. Acknowledgements

The author is greatfully acknowledge the review of the chapter by professor Gábor Nagy and excellent technical assistance of Ágnes Siki to find all necessary data of the references.

7. References

Ainamo, J. & Bay, I. (1975). Problems and proposals for recording gingivitis and plaque, *Int Dent J* 25(4): 229-235.

Alacam, A., Ulusu, T., Bodur, H., Oztas, N. & Oren, M. C. (1996). Salivary and urinary fluoride levels after 1-month use of fluoride-releasing removable appliances, *Caries Res* 30(3): 200-203.

Al Maaltah, E. F., Adeyemi, A. A., Higham, S. M., Pender, N. & Harrison, J. E. (2011). Factors affecting demineralization during orthodontic treatment: a post-hoc analysis of RCT recruits, *Am J Orthod Dentofacial Orthop* 139(2): 181-191.

Altinova, Y. B., Alacam, A., Aydin, A. & Sanisoglu, S. Y. (2005). Evaluation of a new intraoral controlled fluoride release device, *Caries Res* 39(3): 191-194.

Amaechi, B. T.(2009). Emerging technologies for diagnosis of dental caries: The road so far, *J Appl Phys* 105(10):an:102047

Anderson, G. B., Bowden, J., Morrison, E. C. & Caffesse, R, G. (1997). Clinical effects of chlorhexidine mouthwashes on patients undergoing orthodontic treatment, *Am J Orthod Dentofac Orthop* 111(6): 606-612.

Anderson, M. H., Bales, D .J. & Omnell, K. A. (1993). Modern management of dental caries: the cutting edge is not the dental bur, *J Am Dent Assoc* 124(6): 36-44.

Arends, J. & Schuthof, J. (1975). Fluoride content in human enamel after fluoride application and washing: An in vitro study, *Caries Res* 9(5): 363-372.

Artun, J. (1984). Caries and periodontal reactions associated with long-term use of different types of bonded lingual retainers, *Am J Orthod Dentofac Orthop* 86(2): 112-118.

Artun, J. & Brobakken, BO. (1986). Prevalence of carious white spots after orthodontic treatment with multibonded appliances, *Eur J Orthod* 8(4): 229-234.

Attin, T., Hartmann, O., Hilgers, R. D. & Hellwig, E. (1995). Fluoride retention of incipient enamel lesions after treatment with a calcium fluoride varnish in vivo, *Arch Oral Biol* 40(3): 169-174.

Autio-Gold, J. (2008). The role of chlorhexidine in caries prevention, *Oper Dent* 33(6): 710-716.

Axelsson, P. (1991). A four-point scale for selection of caries risk patients, based on salivary S. mutans levels and plaque formation rate index, In: *Risk Markers for Oral Diseases*, N. Johnson, (Ed), 158-170, Cambridge University Press, ISBN 9780521375634, London, England

Axelsson, P. (1999). Other caries preventive factors. Dietary control, In: *An introduction to risk prediction and preventive dentistry*, P. Axelsson (Ed.) 101-102, Quintessence Publishing Co Inc,. ISBN 0-86-715-361-X, Berlin, Germany

Axelsson, P. (2000). Etiologic factors involved in dental caries, In: *Diagnosis and Risk: Prediction of Dental Caries*, P. Axelsson (Ed.) 1-42, ISBN0-86715-362-8, Quintessence Publishing Co Inc., Chicago, USA

Babacan, H., Sokucu, O., Marakoglu, I., Ozdemir, H. & Nalcaci, R. (2011). Effect of fixed appliances on oral malodor, *Am J Orthod Dentofac Orthop* 139(3): 351-355.

Banks, P. A., Chadwick, S. M., Ascher-McDade, C. & Wright, J. L. (2000). Fluoride-releasing elastomerics - a prospective controlled clinical trial, *Eur J Orthod* 22(4): 401-407.

Banoczy, J., Szoke, J., Kertesz, P., Toth, Z., Zimmermann, P. & Gintner Z. (1989). Effect of amine fluoride stannous fluoride-containing toothpaste and mouth-rinsings on dental plaque, gingivitis, plaque and enamel f-accumulation, *Caries Res* 23(4): 284-288.

Batoni, G., Pardini, M., Giannotti, A., Ota, F., Giuca, M. R., Gabriele, M., Campa, M. & Senesi, S. (2001). Effect of removable orthodontic appliances on oral colonisation by mutans streptococci in children, *Eur J Oral Sci* 109(6): 388-392.

Benson, P. (2008). Evaluation of white spot lesions on teeth with orthodontic brackets, *Semin Orthod* 14(3): 200-208.

Benson P. E, Parkin N, Millett D. T, Dyer F. E, Vine, S. & Shah A. (2004). Fluorides for the prevention of white spots on teeth during fixed brace treatment, *Cochrane Database Syst Rev* (3): CD003809.

Bickel, M. & Geering, A. H. (1982). Zur bakteriellen Besiedelung der Prothesenbasis, *Schweiz Monatsschr Zahnheilkd* 92(9): 741-745.

Bishara, S. E. & Ostby, A. W. (2008). White spot lesions: formation, prevention, and treatment, *Semin Orthod* 14(3): 174-182.

Bittencourt, M. A. V. & Machado, A. W. (2010). An overview of the prevalence of malocclusion in 6 to 10 –year-old children in Brazil, *Dental Press Orthod* 15(6): 113-22.

Boersma, J. G., van der Veen, M. H., Lagerweij, M. D., Bokhout, B. & Prahl-Andersen, B. (2005). Caries prevalence measured with QLF after treatment with fixed orthodontic appliances: influencing factors, *Caries Res* 2005, 39(1): 41-47.

Boyd, R.L. (2001). Orthodontic consideration during orthodontic treatment, *In: Textbook of orthodontics*, Bishara S. E. (Ed.), 442-452, WB Saunders Company, ISBN 0-7216-8289-8, Philadelphia, USA

Boyd, R. L., Leggott, P. J., Quinn, R. S., Eakle, W. S. & Chambers, D. (1989). Periodontal implications of orthodontic treatment in adults with reduced or normal periodontal tissues versus those of adolescents, *Am J Orthod Dentofac Orthop* 96(3): 191-198.

Boyd, R. L. & Baumrind, S. (1992). Periodontal considerations in the use of bonds or bands on molars in adolescents and adults, *Angle Orthod* 62(2): 117-126.

Brochner, A., Christensen, C., Kristensen, B., Tranæus, S., Karlsson, L., Sonnesen, L. & Twetman, S. (2011). Treatment of post-orthodontic white spot lesions with casein phosphopeptide-stabilised amorphous calcium phosphate, *Clin Oral Investig* 15(3): 369-373.

Buckley, L. A. (1980). The relationships between irregular teeth, plaque, calculus and gingival disease. A study of 300 subjects, *Br Dent J* 148(3): 67-69.

Cahen, . M., Frank, R. M., Turlot, J. C. & Jung, M. T. (1982). Comparative unsupervised clinical-trial on caries inhibition effect of monofluorophosphate and amine fluoride dentifrices after 3 years in Strassbourg, France, *Community Dent Oral Epidemiol* 10(5): 238-241.

Castellano, J. B. & Donly, K. J. (2004). Potential remineralization of demineralized enamel after application of fluoride varnish, *Am J Dent* 17(6): 462-464.

Chadwick, B. L., Roy, J., Knox, J. & Treasure, E. T. (2005). The effect of topical fluorides on decalcification in patients with fixed orthodontic appliances: A systematic review, *Am J Orthod Dentofac Orthop* 128(5): 601-606.

Chapman, J. A., Roberts, W. E., Eckert, G. J., Kula, K. S. & González-Cabezas, C. (2010). Risk factors for incidence and severity of white spot lesions during treatment with fixed orthodontic appliances, *Am J Orthod Dentofacial Orthop* 138(2):188-194.

Chaussain, C., Opsahl Vital, S., Viallon, V., Vermelin, L., Haignere, C., Sixou, M. & Lasfargues. J. J. (2010). Interest in a new test for caries risk in adolescents undergoing orthodontic treatment, *Clin Oral Investig* 14(2): 177-185.

Chen, W. C., Zawacki, S. J., Nancollas, G. H. & White, D. J. (1985). Constant composition remineralisation of early carious lesions in bovine enamel, *J Dent Res* 64(Spec. iss.): 301-301.

Chu, C. H. & Lo, E. C. M. (2006). A review of sodium fluoride varnish, *General Dentistry* 54(4): 247-253.

Chung, C. H., Cuozzo, P. T. & Mante, F. K. (1999). Shear bond strength of a resin-reinforced glass ionomer cement: An in vitro comparative study, *Am J Orthod Dentofac Orthop* 115(1): 52-54.

Ciuffolo, F., Manzoli, L., D'Attilio, M., Tecco, S., Muratore, F., Festa, F. & Romano, F. (2005). Prevalence and distribution by gender of occlusal characteristics in a sample of Italian secondary school students: a cross-sectional study, *Eur J Orthod* 27(6): 601-606.

Croll, T. P. & Bullock, G. A. (1994). Enamel microabrasion for removal of smooth surface decalcification lesions, *J Clin Orthod* 28(6): 365-370.

Crossman, C. C. (1981). Salivary lactobacillus counts in the prediction of caries activity, *Community Dent Oral Epidemiol* 9(4): 182-190.

de Bruyn, H. & Arends, J. (1987). Fluoride varnishes--a review, *J Biol Buccale* 15(2): 71-82.

Dean, H. T. (1938). Endemic fluorosis and its relation to dental caries, *Public Health Rep* 53(33): 1443-1452.

Derks, A., Katsaros, C., Frencken, J. E., van't Hof, M. A. & Kuijpers-Jagtman, A. M. (2004). Caries-inhibiting effect of preventive measures during orthodontic treatment with fixed appliances. A systematic review, *Caries Res* 38(5): 413-420.

Dharmaraj, S. (2011). RT-PCR: The basics [Internet] Applied Biosystems [cited: 2011.08.22.] Available from: http://www.ambion.com/techlib/basics/rtpcr/index.html

Diamanti-Kipioti, A., Gusberti, F. A. & Lang, N. P. (1987). Clinical and microbiological effects of fixed orthodontic appliances, *J Clin Periodontol* 14(6): 326-333.

Diedrich, P. (1989). Keimbesiedlung und verschiedene Reinigungsverfahren kieferorthopadischer Gerate, *Fortschr Kieferorthop* 50(3): 231-239.

Dijkman, A. G., de Boer, P. & Arends, J. (1983). In vivo investigation on the fluoride content in and on human enamel after topical applications, *Caries Res* 17(5): 392-402.

Dijkman, T. G. & Arends, J. (1988). The role of 'CaF2-like' material in topical fluoridation of enamel in situ, *Acta Odontol Scand* 46(6): 391-397.

Donly, K. J. & Sasa, I. S. (2008). Potential remineralization of postorthodontic demineralized enamel and the use of enamel microabrasion and bleaching for esthetics, *Semin Orthod* 14(3): 220-225.

Emilson, C. G. (1981). Effect of chlorhexidine gel treatment on streptococcus mutans population in human saliva and dental plaque, *Scand J Dent Res* 89(3): 239-246.

Featherstone, J. D. (2003). The caries balance: Contributing factors and early detection, *J Calif Dent Assoc* 31(2): 129-133.

Featherstone, J. D. B. (2006). Delivery challenges for fluoride, chlorhexidine and xylitol, *BMC Oral Health* 6 (SUPPLEMENTUM 1): S8

Featherstone, J. D., Domejean-Orliaguet, S., Jenson, L., Wolff, M. & Young, D. A. (2007). Caries risk assessment in practice for age 6 through adult, *J Calif Dent Assoc* 35(10): 703-713.

Fischer, C., Lussi, A. & Hotz, P. (1995). Kariostatische Wirkungsmechanismen der Fluoride. Eine Ubersicht, *Schweiz Monatsschr Zahnmed* 105(3): 311-317.

Franke, W., Kuenzel, W., Treide, A. & Bluethner, K. (1977). Karieshemmung durch aminfluorid nach 7 jahren kollektiv angeleiteter mundhygiene, *Stomat DDR* 27(1): 13-16

Frazier, M. C., Southard, T. E. & Doster, P. M. (1996). Prevention of enamel demineralization during orthodontic treatment: An in vitro study using pit and fissure sealants. *Am J Orthod Dentofac Orthop* 110(5): 459-465.

Freundorfer, A., Purucker, P. & Miethke, R.R. (1993). Kieferorthopädische Behandlungen können ohne professionelle Mundhygiene zu dauerhaften Veränderungen der subgingivalenPlaqueflora führen, *Prakt Kieferorthop* 7(3): 187-200.

Friedman, M., Harari, D., Raz, H., Golomb, G. & Brayer, L. (1985). Plaque inhibition by sustained-release of chlorhexidine from removable appliances, *J Dent Res* 64(11): 1319-1321.

Fox, C.H. (1992). New considerations in the prevalence of periodontal disease. New considerations in the prevalence of periodontal disease, *Curr Opin Dent* 2: 5-11.

Gabris, K., Marton, S. & Madlena, M. (2006). Prevalence of malocclusions in Hungarian adolescents, *Eur J Orthod* 28(5): 467-470.

Geiger, A. M. (2001). Malocclusion as an etiologic factor in periodontal disease: a retrospective essay, *Am J Orthod Dentofacial Orthop* 120(2): 112-115.

Geiger, A. M., Wasserman, B. H. & Turgeon, L. R. (1974). Relationship of occlusion and periodontal disease. 8. Relationship of crowding and spacing to periodontal destruction and gingival inflammation, *J Periodontol* 45(1): 43-49.

Geiger, A. M., Gorelick, L., Gwinnett, A. J. & Griswold, P. G. (1988). The effect of a fluoride program on white spot formation during orthodontic treatment, *Am J Orthod Dentofac Orthop* 93(1): 29-37.

Genco, R.J (1996). Current view of risk factors for periodontal diseases, *J Periodontol* 67 (10 Suppl): 1041-1049.

Gerardu, V. A. M., Buijs, M, van Loveren, C. & ten Cate, J. M. (2007). Plaque formation and lactic acid production after the use of amine fluoride/stannous fluoride mouthrinse, *Eur J Oral Sci* 115(2): 148-52.

Gorelick, L., Geiger, A. M. & Gwinnett, A. J. (1982). Incidence of white spot formation after bonding and banding, *Am J Orthod Dentofac Orthop* 81(2): 93-98.

Gwinnett, A. J. & Ceen, RF. (1979). Plaque distribution on bonded brackets - scanning microscope study, *Am J Orthod Dentofac Orthop* 75(6): 667-677.

Hastreiter RJ. (1989). Is 0.4% stannous fluoride gel an effective agent for the prevention of oral diseases, *J Am Dent Assoc* 118(2): 205-208.

Heintze, S. D., Jost-Brinkmann, P. G., Finke, C. & Miethke, R, R. (1999). *Oral health for the orthodontic patient*, 25-43, 111-128, Quinessence publishing Co Inc, ISBN 0-86715-295-8, Chicago, USA

Helm, S. & Petersen, P. E. (1989a). Causal relation between malocclusion and caries, *Acta Odontol Scand* 47(4): 217-221.

Helm, S. & Petersen, P. E. (1989b). Causal relation between malocclusion and periodontal health, *Acta Odontol Scand* 47(4): 223-228.

Herzberg, M. C. & Meyer, M. W. (1996). Effects of oral flora on platelets: possible consequences in cardiovascular disease, *J Periodontol* 67(10 Suppl): 1138-1142.

Hicks, M. J., Silverstone, L. M. & Flaitz, C. M. (1984). A scanning electron microscopic and polarized light microscopic study of acid-etching of caries-like lesions in human tooth enamel treated with sodium fluoride in vitro, *Arch Oral Biol* 29(10): 765-772.

Hollender, L. & Rönnerman, A. (1978). Proximal caries progression in connection with orthodontic treatment, Swed Dent J 2(5): 153-160.

Hotz, P. R. (1982). Prävention von Karies und Gingivitis bei der kieferorthopädischen Behandlung, Schweiz Monatsschr Zahnheilkd. 92(Spec No): 880-888.

Huizinga, E. D., Ruben, J. & Arends, J. (1990). Effect of an antimicrobial-containing varnish on root demineralization in situ, Caries Res 24(2): 130-132.

Huser, M. C,, Baehni, P. C. & Lang, R. (1990). Effects of orthodontic bands on microbiologic and clinical parameters, Am J Orthod Dentofac Orthop 97(3): 213-218.

Ingervall, B. (1962). The influence of orthodontic appliances on caries frequency, Odontol Revy 13(2): 175-190.

Jeffcoat, M.K. & McGuire, M. & Newman, M.G. (1997). Evidence-based periodontal treatment. Highlights from the 1996 World Workshop in Periodontics, J Am Dent Assoc 128(6): 713-724.

Jensen, D. & Bratthall, D. (1989). A new method for the estimation of mutans streptococci in human-saliva, J Dent Res 68(3): 468-471.

Katz, R. V. (1978). An epidemiologic study of the relationship between various states of occlusion and the pathological conditions of dental caries and periodontal disease, J Dent Res 57(3): 433-439.

Klock, B. & Krasse, B. (1979). Comparison between different methods for prediction of caries activity, Scand J Dent Res 87(2): 129-139.

Kneist, S., Laurisch, L., Heinrich-Weltzien, R. & Stosser, L. (1998). A modified mitis salivarius medium for a caries diagnostic test, J Dent Res 77(Spec. Issue B):970-970. an. 2712.

Kohler, B. & Bratthall, D. (1979). Practical method to facilitate estimation of streptococcus-mutans levels in saliva, J Clin Microbiol 9(5): 584-588.

Krasse, B. (1988). Biological factors as indicators of future caries, Int Dent J 38(4): 219-225.

Kristoffersson, K., Grondahl, HG. & Bratthall, D. (1985). The more streptococcus-mutans, the more caries on approximal surfaces, J Dent Res 64(1): 58-61.

Kuusela, S., Honkala, E. & Rimpelä, A. (1996). Toothbrushing frequency between the ages of 12 and 18 years - longitudinal prospective studies of Finnish adolescents, Community Dent Health 13(1): 34-39.

Künzel, W., Franke, W. & Treide, A. (1977). Klinisch-röntgenologische Parallelüberwachung einer Längsschnittstudie zum Nachweis der Karieshemmenden Effektivität 7 Jahre lokal angewandten Aminfluorids im Doppelblindtest, Zahn Mund Kieferheilk 65(6): 626-637.

Lagerweij, M. D., Damen, J. J. M. & Stookey, G. K. (1997). Remineralization of small enamel lesions by fluoride, J Dent Res 76 (Spec Issue): 22-22.

Lang, N. P. & Bragger, U. (1991). Periodontal diagnosis in the 1990s, J Clin Periodontol 18(6): 370-379.

Larmas, M. (1975). A new dip slide method for the counting of salivary lactobacilli, Proc Finn Dent Soc 71(2): 31-35.

Leous, P., Pakhomov, G. & Ramanathan, J. (1995). Effectiveness of toothbrushing with amine fluoride toothpaste in the prevention of caries and periodontal diseases among young adults, WHO, Geneva

Linton, J. L. (1996). Quantitative measurements of remineralization of incipient caries, Am J Orthod Dentofac Orthop 110(6): 590-597.

Loe, H., Von der Fehr, F. R. & Schiott, C. R. (1972). Inhibition of experimental caries by plaque prevention. the effect of chlorhexidine mouthrinses *Scand J Dent Res* 80(1): 1-9.

Lundstrom, F., Hamp, S. E. & Nyman, S. (1980). Systematic plaque control in children undergoing long-term orthodontic treatment, *Eur J Orthod* 2(1): 27-39.

Lundstrom, F., & Krasse, B. (1987). Streptococcus mutans and lactobacilli frequency in orthodontic patients; the effect of chlorhexidine treatments, *Eur J Orthod* 9(1): 109-116.

Madlena, M., Vitalyos, G., Marton, S. & Nagy, G. (2000). Effect of chlorhexidine varnish on bacterial levels in plaque and saliva during orthodontic treatment, *J Clin Dent* 11(2): 42-46.

Madlena, M., Nagy, G., Gabris, K., Marton, S., Keszthelyi G. & Banoczy, J. (2002). Effect of amine fluoride toothpaste and gel in high risk groups of Hungarian adolescents: Results of a longitudinal study, *Caries Res* 36(2): 142-146.

Madlena, M., Dombi, C., Gintner, Z. & Banoczy, J. (2004) Effect of amine fluoride/stannous fluoride toothpaste and mouthrinse on dental plaque accumulation and gingival health, *Oral Dis* 10(5): 294-297.

Madlena, M., Banoczy, J., Gotz, G., Szadeczky, B., Marton, S. & Nagy, G. (2009). Effects of Amine Fluoride/Stannous Fluoride Products on Plaque accumulation and Gingival Health in Orthodontic patients, *Caries Res* 43(3): 210-210. an. 86

Marinho, V. C., Higgins, J. P., Logan, S. & Sheiham, A. (2002). Fluoride varnishes for preventing dental caries in children and adolescents, *Cochrane Database Syst Rev (Online)* (3): CD002279

Marthaler, T. M. (1968). Caries-inhibition after seven years of unsupervised use of an amine fluoride dentifrice, *Br Dent J* 124(11): 510-515.

Marthaler, T. M. (1974). Caries-inhibition by an amine fluoride dentifrice results after 6 years in children with low caries activity, *Helv Odontol Acta* 18(Suppl 8): 35-44.

Marthaler, T. M. (1988). Clinical cariostatic effects of various fluoride methods and programs, In: *Fluoride in Dentistry*, Ekstrand, J., Fejerskov, O. & Silverstone, L. M. (Eds.), 252-275, Munksgaard, ISBN 9788716099624, Copenhagen, Denmark

Marthaler, T. M., Konig, K. G. & Muhlemann, H. R. (1970). The effect of a fluoride gel used for supervised toothbrushing 15 or 30 times per year, *Helv Odontol Acta* 14(2): 67-77.

Marton, S., Nagy, G., Gabris, K., Banoczy, J. & Madlena, M. (2008). Logistic regression analysis of oral health data in assessing the therapeutic value of amine fluoride containing products, *OHDMBSC* 7(4): 26-29.

Matthijs, S. & Adriaens, P. A. (2002). Chlorhexidine varnishes: a review, *J Clin Periodontol* 29(1): 1-8.

Mellberg, J. R., Laakso, P. V. & Nicholson, C. R. (1966). The acquisition and loss of fluoride by topically fluoridated human tooth enamel, *Arch Oral Biol* 11(12): 1213-1220.

Mengel, R., Wissing, E., Schmitz Habben, A. & Flores de Jacoby, L. (1996). Comparative study of plaque and gingivitis prevention by AmF/SnF2 and NaF - A clinical and microbiological 9-month study, *J Clin Periodontol* 23(4): 372-378.

Meurman, J. H. (1988). Ultrastructure, growth, and adherence of streptococcus mutans after treatment with chlorhexidine and fluoride, *Caries Res* 22(5): 283-287.

Miethke, R. R. & Newesely, H. (1988). Continuous fluoride release from removable appliances, *J Clin Orthod* 22(8): 490-491.

Miller, J. & Hobson, P. (1961). The relationship between malocclusion, oral cleanliness, gingival conditions and dental caries in school children, *Br Dent J* 111(2): 43-52.

Millett, D. T., Nunn, J. H., Welbury, R. R. & Gordon, P. H. (1999). Decalcification in relation to brackets bonded with glass ionomer cement or a resin adhesive, *Angle Orthod* 69(1): 65-70.

Mirth, D. B. (1980). The use of controlled and sustained release agents in dentistry: A review of applications for the control of dental caries, *Pharmacol Ther Dent* 5(3-4), 59-67.

Mitchell, L. (1992). Decalcification during orthodontic treatment with fixed appliances--an overview, *Br J Orthod* 19(3): 199-205.

Mizrahi, E. (1982). Enamel demineralization following orthodontic treatment, *Am J Orthod Dentofac Orthop* 82(1): 62-67.

Mtaya, M., Brudvik, P. & Astrom, A. N. (2009). Prevalence of malocclusion and its relationship with socio-demographic factors, dental caries, and oral hygiene in 12- to 14-year-old Tanzanian schoolchildren, *Eur J Orthod* 31(5): 467-476.

Muhler, J. C. (1970). Dental caries--orthodontic appliances--SnF$_2$, *J Dent Child* 37(3): 218-221.

Mühlemann, H. R., Schmid, H. S. & Konig, K. G. (1957) Enamel solubility reduction studies with inorganic and organic fluorides, *Helv Odont Acta* 1: 23-33.

Nagy, G., Banoczy, J., Gotz, G., Szadeczky, B., Marton, S. & Madlena, M. (2010). Effects of amine fluoride/stannous fluoride products on oral microflora in orthodontic patients, *Caries Res* 44(3): 200-200. n.73

Newbrun, E. (1992). Current regulations and recommendations concerning water fluoridation, fluoride supplements, and topical fluoride agents, *J Dent Res* 71(5), 1255-1265.

Newbrun, E., Matsukubo, T., Hoover, C. I., Graves, R. C., Brown, A. T., Disney, J. A. & Bohannan, H. M. (1984). Comparison of 2 screening-tests for streptococcus mutans and evaluation of their suitability for mass screenings and private-practice, *Community Dent Oral Epidemiol* 12(5): 325-331.

Nicholson, J. W. (2006). Biologic Considerations, In: *Fundamentals of Operative Denistry. A contemporary approach*, Summitt, J. B., Robbins, J. W., Hilton, T. J. & Schwartz, R. S. (Eds.), 2-4, Quintessence Publishing, ISBN: 978-0-86715-452-8, Chicago, USA

Nicolau, B., Marcenes, W., Bartley, M. & Sheiham, A. (2003). A life course approach to assessing causes of dental caries experience: The relationship between biological, behavioural, socio-econornic and psychological conditions and caries in adolescents, *Caries Res* 37(5): 319-326.

Nobile, C. G. A., Pavia, M., Fortunato, L. & Angelillo, I. F. (2007). Prevalence and factors related to malocclusion and orthodontic treatment need in children and adolescents in Italy, *Eur J Public Health* 17(6): 637-641.

Nyvad, B., Machiulskiene, V. & Baelum, V. (1999). Reliability of a new caries diagnostic system differentiating between active and inactive caries lesions, *Caries Res* 33(4): 252-260.

Obersztyn, A. & Kolwinski, K. (1984). Amine fluoride gel in a caries prophylaxis program for soldiers in Poland, *Community Dent Oral Epidemiol* 12(5): 288-291.

Ogaard, B. (1989). Prevalence of white spot lesions in 19-year-olds - a study on untreated and orthodontically treated persons 5 years after treatment, *Am J Orthod Dentofac Orthop* 96(5): 423-427.

Ogaard, B. (1989). Incidence of filled surfaces from 10-18 years of age in an orthodontically treated and untreated group in Norway, *Eur J Orthod* 11(2): 116-119.

Ogaard, B. (2008). White spot lesions during orthodontic treatment: Mechanisms and fluoride preventive aspects, *Semin Orthod* 14(3): 183-193.

Ogaard, B., Gjermo, P. & Rolla, G. (1980). Plaque-inhibiting effect in orthodontic patients of a dentifrice containing stannous fluoride, *Am J Orthod Dentofac Orthop* 78(3):266-272.

Ogaard, B., Rolla, G., & Helgeland, K. (1984). Fluoride retention in sound and demineralized enamel in vivo after treatment with a fluoride varnish (Duraphat), *Scand J Dent Res* 92(3): 190-197.

Ogaard, B., Rolla, G. & Arends, J. (1988). Orthodontic appliances and enamel demineralization. Part 1. Lesion development, *Am J Orthod Dentofac Ortop* 94(1): 68-73.

Ogaard, B., Duschner, H., Ruben, J. & Arends, J. (1996). Microradiography and confocal laser scanning microscopy applied to enamel lesions formed in vivo with and without fluoride varnish treatment, *Eur J Oral Sci* 104(4): 378-383.

Ogaard, B., Bishara, S. E. & Duschner, H. (2004). Enamel effects during bonding –debonding and treatment with fixed appliances, In: *Risk management in orthodontics: experts' guide to malpractice*, Graber, T. M., Eliades, T. & Atanasiou, A. (Eds.), 19-46, Quintessense Publishing Co, ISBN 0-86715-431-4, Chicago, USA

Öhrn K. & Sanz M. (2009). Prevention and therapeutic approach to gingival inflammation, *J Clin Periodontol* 36(Suppl. 1): 20-26.

O'Reilly, M. M. & Featherstone, J. D. B. (1987). Demineralization and remineralization around orthodontic appliances - an in vivo study, *Am J Orthod Dentofac Orthop* 92(1): 33-40.

Ostberg, A., Halling, A. & Lindblad, U. (1999). Gender differences in knowledge, attitude, behavior and perceived oral health among adolescents, *Acta Odontol Scand* 57(4): 231-236.

Ostela, I. & Tenovuo, J. (1990). Antibacterial activity of dental gels containing combinations of amine fluoride, stannous fluoride, and chlorhexidine against cariogenic bacteria, *Scand J Dent Res* 98(1): 1-7.

Oulis C. J. Raadal I. & Markus L, (2009). Guidelines on the use of fluoride in children: an EAPD policy document. European Academy of Paediatric Dentistry (2009). Guidelines on the use of fluoride in children: an EAPD policy document, *Eur Arch Paediatr Dent* 10(3): 129-35.

Patz, J. & Naujoks, R. (1970). Die kariesprophylaktische Wirkung einer aminfluoridhaltigen Zahnpaste bei Jugendlichen nach dreijahrigem unuberwachten Gebrauch, *Dtsch Zahnarztl Z* 25(6): 617-625.

Paraskevas S. & van der Weijden G. A. (2006). A review of the effects of stannous fluoride on gingivitis, *J Clin Periodontol* 33(1): 1-13.

Pessan, J. P., Al-Ibrahim, N. S., Buzalaf, M. A. R. & Toumba, K. J. (2008). Slow-release fluoride devices: A literature review, *J. Appl Oral Sci* 16(4): 238-246.

Petersson, L. G. (1975). *On topical application of fluorides and its inhibiting effect on caries* [Thesis]. University of Lund, Malmö

Petersson, L. G., Edwardsson, S. & Arends, J. (1992). Antimicrobial effect of a dental varnish, in vitro, *Swed Dent J* 16(5): 183-189.

Petersson, L. G. (1993). Fluoride mouthrinses and fluoride varnishes, Caries Res 27(1): 35-42.

Petersson, L. G., Maki, Y., Twetman, S. & Edwardsson, S. (1991). Mutans streptococci in saliva and interdental spaces after topical applications of an antibacterial varnish in schoolchildren, *Oral Microbiol Immunol* 6(5): 284-287.

Pistorius, A., Rockmann, P., Martin, M. & Willershausen B. (2002). Effectiveness of hyaluronic acid (Gengigel (R)) in the therapy of gingivitis, *J Dent Res* 81(Spec. Issue):A453 an: 3694.

Rabe, H., Miethke, RR. & Newesely, H. (1986). Gefüge und Festigkeit von Silberloten für die Kieferorthopädie nach Behandlung mit handelsüblichen "Zahnspangenreinigern", *Dtsch Zahnarztl Z* 41(7):714-719.

Retief, D. H., Harris, B. E. & Bradley, E. L. (1985). In vitro enamel fluoride uptake from topical fluoride agents, *Dent Materials* 1(0). 93 97.

Reynolds, E. C. (1987). The prevention of sub-surface demineralization of bovine enamel and change in plaque composition by casein in an intra-oral model, *J Dent Res* 66(6): 1120-1127.

Ringelberg, M. L., Webster, D. B., Dixon, D. O. & Lezotte, D. C. (1979). Caries-preventive effect of amine fluorides and inorganic fluorides in a mouthrinse or dentifrice after 30 months of use, *J Am Dent Assoc* 98(2): 202-208.

Rogers, S., Chadwick, B. & Treasure, E. (2010). Fluoride-containing orthodontic adhesives and decalcification in patients with fixed appliances: A systematic review, *Am J Orthod Dentofac Orthop* 138(4): 390.e1-8.

Rodd, H. D. & Davidson, L. E. (1997). The aesthetic management of severe dental fluorosis in the young patient, *Dent Update* 24(10): 408-411.

Rolla, G. & Saxegaard, E. (1990). Critical evaluation of the composition and use of topical fluorides, with emphasis on the role of calcium fluoride in caries inhibition, *J Dent Res* 69(SPEC. ISS. FEB.): 780-785.

Rolla, G., Ogaard, B. & Cruz, R. A. (1991). Clinical effect and mechanism of cariostatic action of fluoride-containing toothpastes: A review, *Int Dent J* 41(3): 171-174.

Sakki, T. K., Knuuttila, M. L. E. & Anttila, SS. (1998). Lifestyle, gender and occupational status as determinants of dental health behavior, *J Clin Periodontol* 25(7): 566-570.

Sangamesh, B. & Amitabh, K. (2011) Iatrogenic effects of orthodontic treatment - Review on white spot lesions, *IJSER* 2(5): 1-16.

Schlagenhauf, U., Tobien, P. & Engelfried, P. (1989). Der Einfluss kieferorthopädischer Behandlung auf Parameter des individuellen Kariesrisikos, *Dtsch Zahnarztl Z* 44(10): 758-760.

Schmid, H. F. (1964). Ein neues tauchieringsmittel mit besondres lang anhalten dem intensivem Fluoriderungseffekt, *Stoma* 17: 71-75.

Schmid H. (1983). Chemie und Oberflächenwirkungen der Aminfluoride, *Dtsch Zahnärztl Z*; 38 (Suppl. 1): S9-13.

Segura, A., Donly, K. J. & Wefel, J. S. (1997a). The effects of microabrasion on demineralization inhibition of enamel surfaces, *Quintessence Int* 28(7): 463-466.

Segura, A., Donly, K. J., Wefel, J. S. & Drake, D. (1997b). Effect of enamel microabrasion on bacterial colonization, *Am J Dent* 10(6): 272-274.

Shannon, I. L. & West, D. C. (1979). Prevention of decalcification in orthodontic patients by daily self-treatment with 0.4% SnF2 gel, *Pediatr Dent* 1(2): 101-102.

Shen, C. & Autio-Gold, J. (2002). Assessing fluoride concentration uniformity and fluoride release from three varnishes, *J Am Dent Assoc* 133(2): 176-182.

Shern, R. J., Duany, L. F., Senning, R. S. & Zinner, D. D. (1976). Clinical-study of an amine fluoride gel and acidulated phosphate fluoride gel, *Community Dent Oral Epidemiol* 4(4): 133-136.

Silva, R. G. & Kang, D. S. (2001). Prevalence of malocclusion among Latino adolescents, *Am J Orthod Dentofac Orthop* 119(3): 313-315.

Silness, J. & Loe, H. (1964). Periodontal disease in pregnancy. II. correlation between oral hygiene and periodontal condition, *Acta Odontol Scand* 22(1): 121-135.

Skjorland, K. K. (1973). Plaque accumulation on different dental filling materials, *Scand J Dent Res* 81(7): 538-542.

Socransky, S. S. (1968). Caries-susceptibility tests, *Ann NY Acad Sci* 153(1): 137-146.

Southard, T. E., Cohen, M. E., Ralls, S. A. & Rouse, L. A. (1986). Effects of fixed-appliance orthodontic treatment on DMF indices, *Am J Orthod Dentofac Orthop* 90 (2): 122-126.

Slavkin, H. C. (1997). First encounters: transmission of infectious oral diseases from mother to child, *J Am Dent Assoc* 128(6): 773-778.

Stahl, F. & Grabowski, R. (2004). Malocclusion and caries prevalence: is there a connection in the primary and mixed dentitions?, *Clin Oral Invest* 8(2): 86-90.

Staley, R. N. (2008). Effect of fluoride varnish on demineralization around orthodontic brackets, *Semin Orthod* 14(3): 194-199.

Stecksen-Blicks, C. (1985). Salivary counts of lactobacilli and streptococcus mutans in caries prediction, *Scand J Dent Res* 93(3): 204-212.

Sudjalim, T. R., Woods, M. G. & Manton, D. J. (2006). Prevention of white spot lesions in orthodontic practice: A contemporary review, *Aust Den J* 51(4): 284-289.

Szoke, J. & Kozma, M. (1989). Ergebnisse einer dreijährigen Untersuchung über Zähneputzen mit einem Aminfluorid-Gelee, *Oralprophylaxe* 11(4): 137-143.

Ten Cate, J. M. & Arends, J. (1980). Remineralization of artificial enamel lesions in vitro: III. A study of the deposition mechanism, *Caries Res* 14(6): 351-358.

Thilander, B., Pena, L., Infante, C., Parada, S. S. & De Mayorga, C. (2001). Prevalence of malocclusion and orthodontic treatment need in children and adolescents in Bogota, Colombia. An epidemiological study related to different stages of dental development, *Eur J Orthod* 23(2): 153-167.

Todd, M. A., Staley, R. N., Kanellis, M. J., Donly, K. J. & Wefel, J. S. (1999). Effect of a fluoride varnish on demineralization adjacent to orthodontic brackets, *Am J Ortod Dentofacial Ortop* 116(2): 159-167.

Toumba, K. J. (1996). *In vivo and in vitro evaluation of a slow release fluoride glass for prevention of dental caries in high risk children* [Thesis], University of Leeds, Leeds.

Tranæus, S., Al-Khateeb, S., Björkman, S., Twetman, S. & Angmar-Månsson, B. (2001). Application of quantitative light-induced fluorescence to monitor incipient lesions in caries-active children. A comparative study of remineralisation by fluoride varnish and professional cleaning, *Eur J Oral Sci* 109(2): 71-75.

Twetman, S. & Petersson, L. G. (1997). Effect of different chlorhexidine varnish regimens on mutans streptococci levels in interdental plaque and saliva, *Caries Res* 31(3): 189-193.

Twetman, S., Skold-Larsson, K. & Modeer, T. (1999). Fluoride concentration in whole saliva and separate gland secretions after topical treatment with three different fluoride varnishes, *Acta Odontol Scand* 57(5): 263-266.

Uysal, T., Amasyali, M., Ozcan, S., Koyuturk, A. E. & Sagdic, D. (2011). Effect of antibacterial monomer-containing adhesive on enamel demineralization around orthodontic brackets: an in-vivo study, *Am J Orthod Dentofac Orthop* 139(5): 650-656.

Vanarsdall, R. J.(2000). Periodontal/orthodontic interrelationships, In: *Orthodontics: Current principles and techniques* Graber, T. M. & Vanarsdall, R. .J. (Eds.), 801-838. Mosby Inc, (Third edition), ISBN 0-8151-9363-7, St Louis, USA

Van Leeuwen, M. P. C., Slot, D. E. & Van Der Weijden, G. A. (2011). Essential oils compared to chlorhexidine with respect to plaque and parameters of gingival inflammation: A systematic review, *J Periodontol* 82(2): 174-194.

Volpe, A. R., Petrone, M. E., De Vizio, W., Davies, R. M. & Proskin, H. M. (1996). A review of plaque, gingivitis, calculus and caries clinical efficacy studies with a fluoride dentifrice containing triclosan and PVM/MA copolymer, *J Clin Dent* 7(Suppl): S1-S14.

Vorhies, A. B., Donly, K. J., Staley, R. N. & Wefel, J. S. (1998). Enamel demineralization adjacent to orthodontic brackets bonded with hybrid glass ionomer cements: An in vitro study, *Am J Orthod Dentofac Orthop* 114(6): 668-674.

Warren, D. P., Henson, H. A. & Chan, J. T. (2000). Dental hygienist and patient comparisons of fluoride varnishes to fluoride gels, *J Dent Hyg* 74(2): 94-101.

Welbury, R. R. & Shaw, L. (1990). A simple technique for removal of mottling, opacities and pigmentation from enamel, *Dent Update* 17(4): 161-163.

Welbury, R. R. & Carter, N. E. (1993). The hydrochloric acid-pumice microabrasion technique in the treatment of post-orthodontic decalcification, *Br J Orthod* 20(3): 181-185.

WHO (1994). *Fluorides and oral health. Report of a WHO Expert Committee on Oral Health Status and Fluoride Use*, WHO, Genf: 1-37. ISBN: 92-4-120846-5

Willmot, D. (2008). White spot lesions after orthodontic treatment, *Semin Orthod* 14(3): 209-219.

Zachrisson, B. U. (1975). Fluoride application procedures in orthodontic practice, current concepts, *Angle Orthod* 45(1): 72-81.

Zachrisson, B. U. & Zachrisson, S. (1971). Caries incidence and oral hygiene during orthodontic treatment, *Scand J Dent Res* 79(6): 394-401.

Zachrisson, B. U. & Zachrisson, S. (1971). Caries incidence and orthodontic treatment with fixed appliances, *Scand J Dent Res* 79(3): 183-192.

Zahradnik, R. T. (1980). Effect of fluoride rinses upon in vitro enamel remineralization, *J Dent Res* 59(6): 1065-1066.

Zickert, I., Emilson, C. G. & Krasse, B. (1982). Effect of caries preventive measures in children highly infected with the bacterium streptococcus-mutans, *Arch Oral Biol* 27(10): 861-868.

Zimmermann, A., Flores de Jacoby, L. & Pan, P. (1993). Gingivitis, plaque accumulation and plaque composition under long-term use of meridol®, *J Clin Periodontol* 20(5): 346-351.

4

3D Facial Soft Tissue Changes Due to Orthodontic Tooth Movement

R.A. Al-Sanea[1], B. Kusnoto[2] and C.A. Evans[2]
[1]Department of Dentistry-Central Region,
National Guards Health Affairs
[2]Department of Orthodontics,
University of Illinois at Chicago
[1]Kingdom of Saudi Arabia
[2]USA

1. Introduction

Two-dimensional (2D) geometric morphometric analysis is the predominant basis for assessment of changes in facial structures resulting from orthodontic or orthognathic surgical treatment. Linear, angular and proportional 2D measurements of the profile are used to assess changes that take place in the three-dimensional (3D) facial soft tissues. However, these methods give little information about frontal soft tissue changes following treatment. Since patients tend to assess their appearance from frontal and three-quarter profile views, measurement of orthodontic outcomes only in the sagittal view as recorded in 2D lateral cephalograms or profile photographs may not be sufficiently informative. Cone Beam Computerized Tomography (CBCT) as well as 3D surface laser head scans offer better frontal and three-quarter profile data for diagnosis, treatment planning and patient education purposes. However, these 3D methods result in large computer files that require large virtual memory and storage media. Moreover, due to lack of normative 3D databases, the 3D images produced can only provide descriptive rather than geometric data of clinical significance. This chapter outlines the current methods used for morphometric assessment of facial soft tissues and their applications and limitations in the field of orthodontics. A simple and accurate method for the assessment of 3D changes occurring in facial soft tissues due to orthodontic tooth movement is explained. Finally, volumetric changes occurring after orthodontic tooth movement due to soft tissue profile advancement or soft tissue profile retraction are outlined.

2. Two-dimensional morphometrics of facial soft tissues

2.1 Two-dimensional imaging

Frontal and lateral photographs and anthropometric measurements along with lateral and frontal cephalometrics are considered the standard records for diagnosis and treatment planning in orthodontic treatment. Two-dimensional geometric morphometrics such as linear, angular and proportional measurements are used to assess changes that take place in facial soft tissues. Research including frontal and lateral photographs has shown that some soft tissue measurements tend to be more reliable than others. In general, frontal measurements are more reliable than lateral ones, and linear measurements are more reliable than angular measurements. Measurements that include subnasale, pogonion, and gnathion tend to be less reliable. Despite the fact that much of the reported evidence in the scientific literature is built around two-dimensional measurements, a substantial amount of information is lacking because:

a. Three-dimensional structures are represented by a set of two-dimensional coordinates. Subject/film/focus geometric relationship could lead to size magnification, distortion, vertical and horizontal displacement in relation to imaging source.

b. Patients tend to assess their appearance from frontal and three quarter profile views, measurement of orthodontic outcomes only in the sagittal view as recorded in 2D lateral cephalograms or profile photographs may not be sufficiently informative. An example of that would be surgical orthognathic patients who can relate to malar region changes or mandibular angle and soft tissue chin changes rather than lip profile and incisor position.

c. For pre-treatment consultation or education sessions, and for discussion purposes, patients tend to describe the soft tissue of the face pointing at vermillion border and philtrum of lips and soft tissue facial folds rather than describing landmarks and linear measurements (Figure 1). The facial folds are skin folds or lines that become accentuated with facial expressions. The most significant factors that contribute to the prominence of the folds are excess skin, skin thinning, excess cheek fat, and ptosis of cheek fat. Many research studies are conducted in the field of plastic and cosmetic surgery on changes that take place in the facial folds with aging and with weight loss or weight gain. Since orthodontic tooth movement contributes to soft tissue profile advancement or retraction, in other words thinning or thickening of soft tissue around the lips as a result of tooth movement, then it would be only practical to borrow these terms for the purpose of patient education and treatment planning in the field of orthodontics.

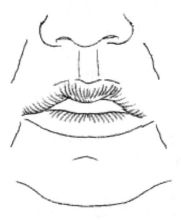

Fig. 1. Facial folds.

2.2 Two-dimensional morphometric analysis of facial soft tissues

When superimposing different faces, a limited number of labeled points on each face, e.g., the tip of the nose, corner of the eye and less prominent points on the cheek must be located precisely (Farkas, 1987). Linear and angular measurements between the landmarks provide useful measurements for comparison. The number of reported manually labeled landmarks varies, but usually ranges from 50 to 300 as shown in Figure 2 (O'Toole et al., 1999; Clement & Marks, 2005). Only a correct alignment of all these points allows acceptable comparison between faces, intermediate morphs, a convincing mapping of motion data from the reference or initial treatment image into final treatment image.

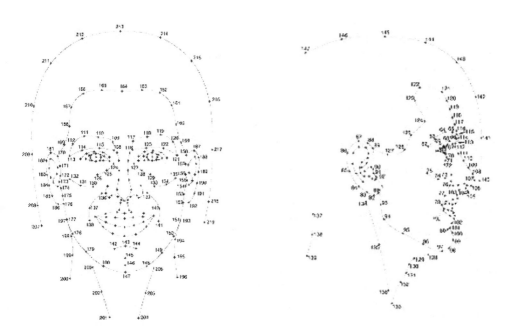

Fig. 2. Soft tissue landmarks of the face (Source: Computer-Graphic Facial Reconstruction, Clement & Murray, eds., p. 114, Figure 6.3).

2.3 Facial soft tissue changes in studies utilizing two-dimensional images

There is controversy in the orthodontic literature regarding the correlation between craniofacial skeletal and soft-tissue profile form (Denis & Speidel, 1987; Bloom, 1961; Burke, 1983; Savara, 1965). For instance, although stereophotogrammetric (Savara, 1965; Burke, 1983; Peck & Peck, 1995), computed tomographic (Marsh & Vannier, 1983; Moss et al., 1987) and cephalometric studies (Riedel, 1950; Tweed, 1944) have indicated soft-tissue profile form is markedly influenced by orthodontic tooth movement and or orthognathic surgery, other studies have suggested the relative independence of the facial soft tissues on the underlying skeletal form (Finnoy et al., 1987; Wisth, 1974).

In an attempt to determine the effects of orthodontic treatment on the soft tissue profile of the lips, several studies were conducted to quantify and to predict the relationship between incisor retraction and lip retraction (Bloom, 1961; Rudee, 1964; Garner, 1974; Roos, 1977; Wisth, 1974; Hershey, 1972). With the exception of one study that found a predictable amount of soft tissue changes in response to incisor retraction (Bloom, 1961) the majority of the studies on both growing and non-growing subjects concluded that the large individual variation prevents the accurate prediction of lip response to incisor retraction in any given person.

Some studies pointed that lip structure seems to have an influence on lip response to incisor retraction. Oliver found that patients with thin lips or a high lip strain displayed a significant correlation between incisor retraction and lip retraction, whereas patients with thick lips or low lip strain displayed no such correlation (Oliver, 1982). In addition, Wisth (1974) found that lip response, as a proportion of incisor retraction, decreased as the amount of incisor retraction increased. This seems to indicate that the lips have some inherent support.

Al-Mesad (1998) studied soft tissue changes in extraction and non-extraction orthodontic patients and found that for the most part, the drape of the upper and lower lips was highly correlated to the changes in both upper and lower incisors. Changes in position of upper and lower incisors were found to influence the final position of upper and lower lips after orthodontic treatment in the total sample for both extraction and non-extraction samples. For every millimeter change in the upper incisor tip in the non-extraction group, approximately 0.2 mm of changes in the upper lip and 0.9 mm in the lower lip occurred. Greater changes were observed in individuals with thin upper and lower lips (0.8 mm changes for the upper lip with only 0.6 mm changes for the lower lip).

Bishara et al. (1995) used standardized facial photographs to compare the soft tissue profile changes in persons with Class II, division 1 malocclusions who were treated with either an extraction or non-extraction treatment modalities. The found that: (1) After treatment the upper and lower lips were retracted significantly more in the extraction group compared with the non-extraction group. These differences persisted into retention; (2) Upper lip length increased more among subjects who were treated without extractions; (3) Upper vermilion height in male subjects and the upper and lower vermilion heights in female subjects increased among subjects who were treated without extractions and decreased among subjects who were treated with four first premolar extractions; (4) Nasolabial angle became significantly more obtuse among the female subjects who were treated with four first premolar extractions (Bishara et al., 1995). Similar findings were noted by Kocadereli (2002). On the other hand, Charles Tweed (1944) firmly stated that non-extraction approach would place the teeth in an unstable position in the basal bone leading to unacceptable relapse afterwards.

Paquette et al. (1992) looked at 'borderline' extraction/non-extraction cases 14.5 years out of retention and found that in the long term, the non-extraction patients had profiles that were 2 mm fuller. A similar study (Luppanapornlarp & Johnston, 1993) looked at carefully selected and defined first premolar-extraction cases and non-extraction cases over the same post-retention time frame. The results indicated that the extraction of first premolars tended to flatten the profile by 2-3 mm when compared with non-extraction treatment. Interestingly, the non-extraction patients had the more concave faces post-treatment and this challenges the concept of extractions as part of orthodontic treatment 'dishing the face'. The ability to predict from post-treatment lateral photographs, whether individuals had been treated with or without extractions has been investigated (Boley et al., 1998) The findings indicated a correct response in only 54% of cases - just greater than pure chance.

In a sample of forty adult patients who underwent orthodontic treatment that resulted in either soft tissue profile retraction or soft tissue profile advancement, Al-Sanea, Kusnoto and Evans (Al-Sanea, 2007) studied linear changes occuring in cephalometric soft tissue landmarks: Sn, A, UL, LL, B. Patient selection was based on the following criteria: availability of pre-treatment and post-treatment lateral cephalometric radiographs; availability of acceptable clarity pre-treatment and post-treatment frontal and lateral photographs with lips closed or slightly touching without strain and the patient's head properly oriented in the three planes of space; and absence of facial hair, eye glasses or jewelry. The following criteria were added as part of the study design to minimize undesirable soft tissue facial changes:

1. Any patient with lip incompetence of more than 2 millimeters was excluded as this interfered later on with the morphing procedure in FaceGen™ Modeller 3.1 (Singular Inversions, Toronto, ON, Canada, 2005).
2. Diminished growth with a minimum pre-treatment age of sixteen years for females and eighteen years for males.
3. Absence of craniofacial anomalies or significant skeletal discrepancy.
4. Treatment modalities included fixed appliance therapy with no orthognathic surgical treatment involved in any case.
5. No measurable weight gain or weight loss changes instead of treatment related soft tissue change as determined from interzygomatic width and submental soft tissue which were compared between the pre-treatment and post-treatment frontal photographs after image resizing is carried out in Adobe Photoshop™ software (Adobe System Inc., San Jose, CA, 2005).

In all 2D landmark measurements (Figure 3), a negative soft tissue change was observed in the soft tissue profile retraction group. The opposite was observed in the group that showed advancement of the soft tissue profile. In the profile retraction group, change was the greatest in the upper lip and lower lips (-1.68 and –1.58 mm). Similarly, the most change in the profile advancement group was observed in upper and lower lip and Sn (0.73, 0.85 and 0.86) (Table 1).

In this sample of patients, the overall soft tissue change in the profile retraction group was significantly greater in comparison to the change reported in the profile advancement group in all 2D landmarks (p<0.05). The highest difference in 2D measurements between the two groups was noted in the upper and lower lip (2.40 and 2.42 mms) followed by change at SfB (1.95 mm), followed by change at Sn (1.75 mm) and SfA (1.36 mm). Lack of change at SfA in the soft tissue profile advancement group was the reason why change at SfA was the lowest in comparison to other 2D measurements (Table 2).

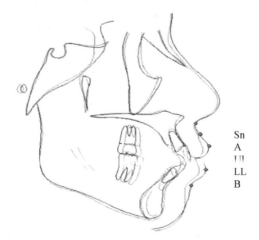

Fig. 3. 2D landmarks of soft tissue profile.

Retraction Group			Advancement Group		
Measurements	N	Mean ± SD (mm)	Measurements	N	Mean ± SD (mm)
2D-Sn	20	-0.89 ± 1.58	2D-Sn	20	0.86 ± 1.65
2D-SfA	20	-0.78 ± 2.14	2D-SfA	20	0.58 ± 1.96
2D-UL	20	-1.68 ± 1.80	2D-UL	20	0.73 ± 2.38
2D-LL	20	-1.58 ± 2.44	2D-LL	20	0.85 ± 2.63
2D-SfB	20	-1.30 ± 2.09	2D-SfB	20	0.65 ± 2.24

* p ≤0.05

Table 1. Means and standard deviations for linear horizontal changes in the soft tissue profile groups.

Measurements	Mean Difference (mm)	Student t -value	p-value*
2D-Sn	-1.75	-3.42	0.001
2D-SfA	-1.36	-2.09	0.044
2D-UL	-2.40	-3.60	0.001
2D-LL	-2.42	-3.02	0.004
2D-SfB	-1.95	-2.84	0.007

* p ≤0.05

Table 2. Comparison of 2D measurements of soft tissue profile retraction and advancement groups.

3. Three-dimensional morphometrics of facial soft tissues

3.1 Three-dimensional facial models

The goal of imaging in medicine and dentistry has been to display a patient's anatomic truth. Until now, imaging technology has been largely confined to two dimensions. The development of a 3D digital model of a patient's anatomy would greatly improve our ability to determine different treatment options, to monitor changes over time (the fourth dimension), to predict and display final treatment results, and to measure treatment outcomes more accurately. Lately, computer graphic head modeling has gained wide popularity in the field of plastic and orthognathic surgery for the prediction and simulation of treatment effects. The technique offers great advantages in surgical planning and the prediction of facial deformation. Furthermore, three-dimensional modeling of patient anatomy allows for engineering principles to be applied to such areas as local and general stress analysis of the stomatognathic system, analysis of asymmetry and how it may affect function, TMJ loading and occlusal forces, and reconstruction in oral and maxillofacial surgery. Finally, functional studies on dynamic 3D models will help us to understand the dynamic relationship of the anatomy which orthodontists and maxillofacial surgeons affect everyday in their practices (Quintero et al., 1999; Moss &Linney, 1990; Hatcher & Dial, 1999, Harrell et al., 2002).

3.1.1 Directly acquired three-dimensional facial models

Three-dimensional facial models "3D Facial Model" can be defined as three-dimensional coordinate data of facial soft tissues (Figure 4). Facial models can be acquired directly in 3D format utilizing computed tomograms (CT), including cone-beam tomography, magnetic resonance imaging (MRI), digital radiography, and digital ultrasound. Those techniques involve the use of ionizing radiation with varying degree, and can produce facial models with surface as well as deep data, depending on degree of segmentation.

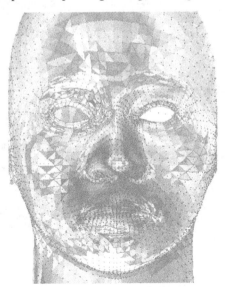

Fig. 4. Three-dimensional facial model.

Other direct techniques for producing 3D facial models, that do not involve the use of ionizing radiation, include stereophotogrammetry and simultaneous image capture from more than one camera source. This approach can produce only surface data or a "3D shell of the face." All of the above mentioned allow for the volumetric registration of the hard and or soft tissue of the craniofacial structures and the face with adequate resolution. The end result is a 3D facial model that can be easily viewed on a computer monitor. However, all the techniques generate huge files that require large virtual memory and storage media.

3.1.2 Manually reconstructed three-dimensional facial models

Facial Models can be reconstructed into 3D format utilizing a variety of 2D or 3D images that are calibrated and merged into a 3D "digital replica" of anatomy. Surface laser scanning can produce multiple 3D images from different angles with a spatial resolution of 0.5 mm (Figure 5). Those images can be manually stitched together, utilizing the scanner software, into a 3D facial model. Similarly, multiple 2D images taken at different views can also be used to construct 3D facial models. In both cases, texture data can be mapped on to the 3D surface which produces a photorealistic 3D model. The main draw back in these settings is that post-processing of the acquired data can significantly alter the dimensions and appearance, particularly with over smoothing. While there have been numerous reports on the use of 3D facial images in evaluation of facial soft tissue changes following orthognathic surgery, these approaches and systems have not been critically validated. The task of validation of these systems for facial imaging is difficult due to the multitude of variables in post-processing and the conditions of image acquisition in the clinic.

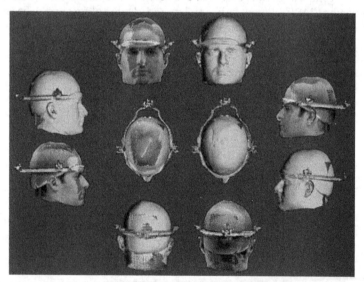

Fig. 5. Different surface laser scans before stitching into one 3D head model. (Source: Computer-Graphic Facial Reconstruction, Clement & Murray, eds., p. 234, Figure 12.9).

Furthermore, all systems suffer from potential for patient movement and alterations of facial expression between the multiple views needed to construct a 3D model of the face. Laser-based systems are a safety concern. While these systems are deemed safe for use with adults, the United State Food and Drug Administration (FDA) has no statement on the safety of laser systems in children, who constitute a majority of the orthodontic and craniofacial treatment group. The light-based imaging systems generally lack the precision of the laser-based systems and suffer from image artifacts due to skin tone, color and reflectance. Additionally, the majority of 3D imaging systems utilize frontal and three-quarter facial views to produce a facial model; however this approach does not provide sufficiently accurate representations of the facial profile. The "profile" view generated from these systems is not a true view of the facial profile, as one would have with a camera positioned from the patient's profile. The generated "profile" can be distorted by several millimeters and lack detail of specific features, especially in the lower face and lips. This deficiency is a significant setback because much of our knowledge of growth and development and treatment outcomes is based upon the profile view.

3.1.3 Mathematically reconstructed three-dimensional facial models

This process involves the use of a framework of anthropometric measurements and texture information that characterize faces in a data set of 3D head scans. Principal Component Analysis (PCA), which is a powerful statistical technique that has found application in fields such as face recognition and image compression where the luxury of graphical representation is not available, can be utilized to analyze patterns of similarities and differences in this data set. After finding patterns in the data, anthropometric measurements and texture information act as geometric constraints for morphing a prototype (i.e., average) 3D facial model. This avarage is then registered on the 2D image and mathematically mapped into a 3D model of the face. A hierarchial algorithm is applied to adjust the model parameters for an optimal 3D reconstruction of the target image. Some imaging software utilize robust mathematical registration and algorithmic methods for the automatic mapping or simulation of faces with varying degree of accuracy depending on the amount of detailed information obtained from the date set. In applying the method to several images of a person, and when more detailed statistics (such as covariance information or exact distributions) are included, the 3D reconstructions can reach almost the quality of laser scans (Blanz & Vetter, 1999). The herarchial modeling technique utilized in software Facegen™ Modeller 3.5 (Singular Inversions, 2009) would serve as a practical, accurate and user friendly interface for the mathematical reconstruction of 3D facial models from readily available 2D images of orthodontic treatments and growth studies.

3.2 Three-dimensional morphometric analysis of facial soft tissue

Many studies were conducted on the evaluation of facial soft tissues utilizing 3D facial models of orthognathic surgical cases. Regardless whether the facial model was a true capture or a reconstructed one, several factors are impeding our understanding of 3D soft tissue changes in the orthodontic/orthognathic field:

- Lack of normative 3D craniofacial databases that are age-, gender-, race-specific for reference purposes in diagnosis and treatment planning.
- Lack of 3D data of facial changes during growth, maturation, and aging.
- Superimposition methods that do not work: Two-dimensional measurements rely solely on manual annotation with landmarks. This procedure is time-consuming and subject to

error in 3D facial models. Three-dimensional models require sophisticated registration mathematics for analysis. The combined robust mathematics in the Euclidean Distance Matrix Analysis (EDMA) and Dense Correspondence Algorithm (DCA) serve as reliable registration methods for 3D models. However, further sophisticated mechanisms such as Thin Spline Plate Analysis (TSP) and Finite Element Analysis (FEA) need to be utilized for comparison of 3D changes between pre treatment and post treatment models.

• The 3D images before, during and after processing require computer processers with large virtual memories, not to mention the large storage and back up needed.

3D Facial Model	Acquired	Manually reconstructed	Mathematically reconstructed
Pros	True replica Of surface anatomy. Deep data as well in Cone Beam CT	Almost true replica of surface anatomy	Surface anatomy with quality similar to surface laser scans, utilizes readily available 2D images, inexpensive method, user friendly, no radiation or laser use
Cons	Radiation exposure in CBCT, light based systems produce image artifacts and potential for patient movement while image capture	Stitching required, over smoothening, computer manipulation, laser use poses safety concerns, potential for patient movement while image capture	Not true capture, Computer manipulation required

Table 3. A comparison between the three different modes of acquisition of 3D facial models.

3.2.1 Three-dimensional methods of registration

3.2.1.1 Euclidean distance matrix analysis (EDMA)

In general, the distance between points   and   in a Euclidean space is given by Weisstein (Weisstein, 1999)

$$d = |x - y| = \sqrt{\sum_{i=1}^{x'} |x_i - y_i|^2}$$

To explain the method of EDMA, let's represent an object by M (K X D) matrix where K is number of landmarks in the object and D is the dimensions, in which these landmarks lie, i.e., a landmark coordinate system (Lele & Richtsmeire, 1991; Lele & Cole, 1995). The form of an object as represented by this collection of landmark coordinates is that characteristic which remains invariant under the group of transformation consisting of rotation (spinning the object on an axis), reflection and translation (moving the object within a given coordinate system). The invariant condition is when the Difference M1, M2 = Diff (M1 R1+1t1, M2 R2+1t2) for any choice of rotation parameters R1, R2 and translation parameters t1, t2. A collection of all K X D matrices that can be obtained by rotation, reflection and translation of M is called an orbit. Under definition of form all matrices in the same orbit represent exactly the same form.

Any object with K landmarks in D dimensions can be represented in an invariant fashion using the vector of distances between all possible pairs of landmarks. This is called the form matrix (Lele & Richtsmeier, 1991). In the Euclidean Distance Matrix Analysis (EDMA) for any two objects with K landmarks, we end up with two form matrices i.e., the vectors of all possible pair wise distances for each one of the objects. One particular description that has been used to outline the difference between these two objects is the vector of the ratios of the corresponding differences, i.e., the form difference matrix (Lele and Richtsmeier, 1991; Lele & Cole, 1995). The important property of this description is that it only depends on the orbits to which the two forms belong, not on the exact locations along these orbits. This overcomes the problem of the lack of the coordinate system for location of change.

3.2.1.2 Finite Element Analysis (FEA)

Three-dimensional face models are described from a mathematical point of view by a huge number of polygons, forming something like a mesh. The nodes of the mesh are the vertices of the polygons. Finite-element scaling analysis can be used to depict clinical changes in terms of allometry (size-related shape-change), and the change in form between an initial configuration and a target configuration can be viewed as a continuous deformation from the initial form, which can be quantified based on major and minor strains (principal strains). If the two strains are equal, the change in form is characterized by a simple increase or decrease in size. However, if one of the principal strains changes in a greater proportion, both size and shape are transformed. The product of the strains indicates a change in size if the result is not equal to 1. For example, a product >1 indicates an increase in size (measured from the base of the mesh of the initial form) equal to the remainder; 1.30 indicates a 30% increase in volume (positive allometry). Similarly, a product of 0.65 indicates a 35% decrease in volume (negative allometry). The products and ratios can be resolved for individual landmarks within the configuration and these can be made linear using a log-linear scale. For ease of interpretation, a pseudocolour-coded scale can be used to provide a graphic display of change in size, as shown in Figure 6 (Singh et al., 2006).

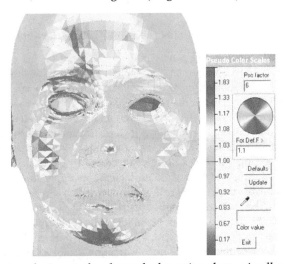

Fig. 6. Finite element analysis pseudocolor scale depecting change in allometry between initial and target 3D facial model.

3.2.1.3 Thin Plate Spline analysis (TPS)

Suppose that all of the specimen landmarks, in the initial stage, are embedded into a thin, 2D, non-deformed, elastic plate. Due to transformation, landmarks will migrate to other new positions (final stage), so the thin-plate will be distorted, that is, all of the points belonging to the thin-plate will be relocated or dragged by landmark movements. TPS is applied to the comparison of forms as a regression mechanism with the requirement that bending energy or smoothness function is minimized. Applying finite element algorithms, it's possible to define an Area Factor, a Deformation Factor and a Principal Axis Direction for any point in the plate after deformation.

3.2.1.4 Dense Correspondence Algorithm (DCA)

For three-dimensional morphometric comparisons of pre-treatment and post-treatment head models, comparisons cannot be carried out unless the models are homologous (having equal number of nodes). Based on the closest point algorithm, the post-treatment meshes will utilize the landmarks from the pre-treatment head model as the basic mesh for the dense correspondence procedure when comparing the pre- to post-treatment head model of the same patient. In the closest point algorithm principle, the two models are aligned utilizing the digitized surface landmarks. The new position of the target vertices that lie in-between the landmarks of the post-treatment model are determined using the Euclidean Distance Matrix Analysis (EDMA) approach. This way the points in the reassembled post-treatment mesh have a one-to-one correspondence with those of the pre-treatment mesh. Finally Thin-Plate Spline analysis is applied. As a result, all of the forms will have the same quantity of nodes, which enables comparison later on (Hutton et al., 2001).

Care should be taken in specifying the greatest distance between homologous landmarks while alignment of the head models. If the distance between a generic landmark of the basic mesh (pre-treatment model) and the surface of any non-basic mesh (post-treatment model) is greater than the parameter specified, then the landmark is definitively discarded.

3.3 Facial soft tissue changes in studies utilizing three-dimensional images

Ismail and Moss (2002) prospectively compared the 2D and the 3D effects on the face of extraction and non-extraction orthodontic treatment in patients with skeletal Class I patterns. They showed, based on cephalometric values, that the nasolabial angle was larger in the extraction group, while the vermilion boarder of the upper lip was forward in comparison to the extraction group at the end of treatment. Differential geometrics and surface shape analysis showed that for the two treatment modalities in the current study, there was a significant difference in the changes in upper lip thickness. The reduction in upper lip thickness in the extraction group was accompanied by a decrease in exposed vermilion. The converse was true for the non-extraction group, which showed an increase in upper lip thickness in the study. Furthermore, the non-extraction group had more convex cheeks and chins by the end of treatment compared to the extraction group. They also pointed an increased concavity of the labiomental fold region by the end of treatment in the extraction group. Faces in the extraction group became relatively more protrusive with treatment. The surface shape analysis technique showed that the cheeks were flatter in the none-extraction group at the start of treatment, but this reversed with time. In the extraction group, the concavity of the labiomental fold increased, while the non-extraction group showed no change in this area.

In a geometric morphometric study on changes in the soft tissue facial profile following orthodontics, Singh et al. (2005) reported a statistically significant difference in the premaxillary region with the non-extraction group being relatively larger in that region by 25%. For the non-extraction group after treatment, localized increases in relative size in the naso-maxillary region size of 25% (p < 0.01) were present. For the extraction group after treatment, a non-significant reduction in relative size of 15% was localized in the putative bicuspid area.

Studies that used FEA to analyze the effect of extraction and non-extraction orthodontic treatment mostly used lateral cephalometrics. Finite elements were constructed using anatomical landmarks in lateral cephalometrics as vertices of the triangular elements and then analysis was carried out as the deformational change needed to produce the final cephalometric radiograph (Lavelle & Carvalho, 1989; Singh et al., 2005). The technique is good as it portrays the change as the amount of strain required to produce the final image. However, the technique utilizes two-dimensional images to portray three-dimensional structures. Therefore, those studies inherit the same limitations associated with studies of two-dimensional data.

Other studies used surface shape analysis to report changes in the face after orthodontic treatment (Ismail & Moss, 2002). They used 3D surface laser scans and compared faces after extraction and non-extraction orthodontic treatment. The experimental design involved description of the shape of the surfaces (i.e., saddle, spherical, dome, ridge, etc). The comparison was carried out mainly to detect how the surface changed in either shape or area. The technique might be useful in terms of comparing three-dimensional data on its own. However, much of our knowledge in growth and development and treatment results are derived from two dimensional landmark measurements of two-dimensional radiographs and photographs.

4. Morphometric analysis of three-dimensional facial models generated utilizing two-dimensional photographs

Much of our knowledge of treatment outcomes and growth and development of facial soft tissues is based on the frontal and profile photographs of patients. It would be greatly advantagous if these readily available images can be data mined into 3D facial models. A simple and accurate technique for the generation of 3D facial models from sets of 2D readily available pre treatment and post treatment photographs is proposed by Al-Sanea, Kusnoto and Evans (Al-Sanea, 2007).

The pretreatment and post-treatment images for each patient are resized by creating a duplicate layer of the post-treatment image in a contrasting balance, and then adjusting the opacity of the created layer to 60-70%. Later on the post-treatment image layer is overlaid on top of the pretreatment image and its size adjusted until a perfect fit on the eyes is achieved.

Three-dimensional head models were constructed using FaceGen™ Modeller 3.1 and 3.5 (Singular Inversions Inc., Toronto, ON, Canada, 2005 and 2009) from the resized frontal and lateral photographs of the same patients where the 2D cephalometric analysis was carried out. Following the recommendations of the software, 11 surface landmarks were digitized on the frontal photographs and 7 landmarks on the lateral photograph. The surface landmark locations suggested by the software are in accordance with facial soft tissue landmarks definitions outlined by Farkas (1987). After landmark digitization the software computes the average face and the mode of variation in its own dataset based on the age, gender, race, and symmetry information specified to it by the operator. Based on this information the software predicts and produces an average head that can be morphed into the patient's head. During the morphing procedure, the software calculates the texture and geometric information in the image and modifies the 3D model accordingly. The three-dimensional image produced is saved in two formats (Facegen: Fg) and (VRML. 97).

A pre treatment and a post-treatment model were generated for each patient. Computer graphic facial analysis was carried out for those models in each patient using Morphostudio™ 3.02.39 (Orthovisage, New York, NY, 2005). First, twelve surface landmarks are digitized on the face of the model (Figure 7) in order to apply the dense correspondence algorithm. The dense correspondence algorithm transforms vertices in the 3D models into homologous landmarks that are easily compared. For consistency and reliability, the surface landmarks were selected in accordance with the surface landmarks already used to generate the 3D model in Facegen™.

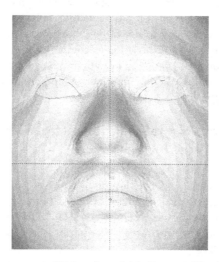

Fig. 7. Landmarks used to generate 3D head model in Facegen™ software as well as apply the dense correspondence algorithm function in Morphostudio™.

The percentage of volume deformation in the post-treatment model (as measured from the base of the mesh of the pretreatment model) was reported through the Finite Element Analysis function of the Morphostudio™ 3.02.39 (Orthovisage, New York, NY, 2005).[30] This is represented in the color-coded graphic display in the software (Figure 6). A total of thirty-four pseudocolor scale measurements were recorded from the surface of the 3D model at different nodes around the lips (Figure 8).

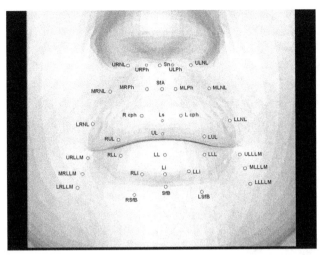

Fig. 8. Landmark areas where psudocolor scale measurements were recorded.

Since the deformation was expressed over a large area around the lips, point measurements at single nodes were not effective. Multiple measurements had to be recorded at different regions around the lips and averaged together in order to report the average volumetric deformation occurring in that region (Figure 9). Measurements were analyzed to determine changes in the soft tissue of the face following orthodontic treatment that resulted in soft tissue profile retraction or soft tissue profile advancement.

As shown in Figure 8, four lateral measurements were recorded on the same horizontal level of Sn at both the nasolabial fold and the philtrum of the upper lip. These measurements were labeled as upper right and left nasolabial fold (URNL, ULNL) and upper right and left philtrum (URPh, ULPh) respectively. Four lateral measurements were recorded on the same horizontal level of SfA on the nasolabial fold and the philtrum of the upper lip. Those measurements were the middle right and left nasolabial and the middle right and left philtrum (MRNL, MLNL, and MRPh, MLPh respectively). Two lateral measurements were also recorded at the junction of the nasolabial fold and the upper lip (lower right nasolabial and lower left nasolabial- LRNL and LLNL). Three measurements were recorded for the upper lip vermillion boarder in the areas of labiale superius (ls) and crista philtri landmark (cph). Three measurements were recorded on the convex surface of the upper lip, two on each side and one in the middle (RUL, MUL, LUL). The same was for the lower lip, two measurements were recorded on each side of the convex surface and one middle measurement was taken (RLL, MLL, LLL). Three measurements right, left and middle were recorded on the lower lip vermilion border (Rli, Mli, Lli). Two measurements were recorded on the labiomental folds on each side of SfB (RSfB, LSfB). Two measurements (URLLM, ULLLM) were recorded on the lateral labiomental folds and fall at the junction of the lateral labiomental folds and the lower lip. Two other measurements on the lateral labiomental folds were recorded and fell on the same horizontal level of Rli, Mli, Lli (MRLLM, MLLLM). Two measurements (RSfB, LSfB) were recorded on the lateral labiomental folds and fell on the same horizontal level of SfB.

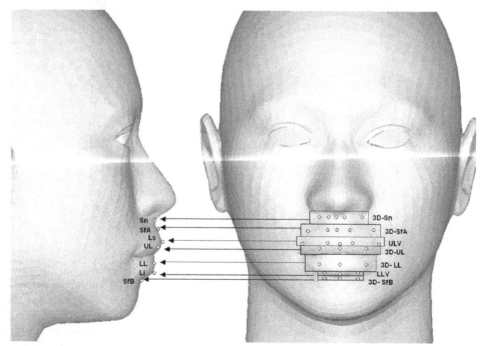

Fig. 9. Averaged 3D measurements.

The percentages of volumetric change were calculated by averaging each five pseudocolor scale measurements on the same horizontal level of each reference landmark. These values were used to report the mean percentage of 3D volumetric change at areas of Sn, SfA, UL, LL, SfB. The averaging procedure for these landmarks is shown in Figure 9.

Furthermore, bilateral measurements at the folds of the face were also averaged. Three bilateral measurements on the right and left nasolabial folds were averaged together denoting change at the nasolabial folds (Right nasolabial fold measurements: URNL, MRNL, LRNL and left nasolabial measurements: ULNL, MLNL, LLNL). All nine measurement enclosed within the philtrum of the upper lip were averaged together (URPh, Sn, ULPh, MRPh, SfA, MLPh, LRPh, Ls, LLPh). Three bilateral vertical measurements on the lateral labiomental folds were averaged together denoting change at the lateral labniomental folds (Right lateral labiomental fold measurements: URLLM, MRLLM, LRLLM and left labiomental fold measurements: ULLLM, MLLLM, LLLLM). These averaged measurements are shown in Figure 10.

Reliability of the FEA method was obtained by recording pseudocolor scale values on different time points for six randomly selected patients and estimating the pair wise correlations among these pseudoscale values. Two-tailed sample Student t-test was calculated to compare the mean measurements in soft tissue profile retraction and soft tissue profile advancement groups at 0.05 level of significance.

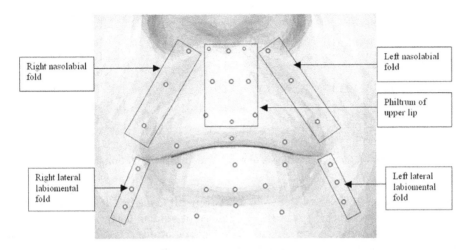

Fig. 10. Average measurements at the folds of the face.

The percentages of volumetric deformation of the surface nodes from the base of the pre-treatment mesh were calculated by averaging the five pseudocolor scale measurements on the same horizontal level of each reference landmark; leading to the mean percentage of volumetric change at areas of Sn, SfA, UL, LL, SfB. Change was the greatest in upper and lower lip measurements in both profile retraction and profile advancement groups. Change in the profile retraction group was the greatest at the upper lip vermilion border (3D-UV), which was 12.47 %. In the soft tissue profile advancement group however, change was greatest at the vermilion border of the lower lip (7.09%). The greatest difference in 3D measurements between the two groups was noted in the vermilion boarder of the upper lip at 15.71% (Tables 4 and 5).

Groups		Retraction	Advancement
Measurements	N	Mean ± SD (%)	Mean ± SD (%)
3D-Sn	20	-7.72 ± 9.51	5.80 ± 9.48
3D-SfA	20	-10.99 ± 7.02	-0.30 ± 12.82
3D-LL	20	-9.92 ± 20.41	4.29 ± 22.91
3D-UL	20	-6.59 ± 14.83	2.00 ± 10.17
3D-LV	20	-2.59 ± 14.65	7.09 ± 17.59
3D-UV	20	-12.47 ± 9.41	3.23 ± 10.81
3D-SfB	20	-8.69 ± 13.49	5.16 ± 10.28

$p \leq 0.05$

Table 4. Means and standard deviations for the percentage of volume deformation in the soft tissue profile groups.

Measurements	Mean Difference	Student t-value	p- value*
3D-Sn	-13.51	-4.50	0.000
3D-SfA	-10.69	-3.27	0.003
3D-UL	-8.56	-2.13	0.040
3D-LL	-14.21	-2.07	0.045
3D-LV	-9.69	-1.89	0.066
3D-UV	-15.71	-4.90	0.000
3D-SfB	-13.86	-3.65	0.001

* p ≤0.05

Table 5. Comparison of 3D measurements of soft tissue profile retraction and advancement groups.

Statistically significant differences were found between soft tissue profile retraction and soft tissue profile advancement groups in the percentage of volume deformation at the facial folds regions. The greatest difference between soft tissue profile retraction and soft tissue profile advancement was noted at the Philtrum (Ph) Where the difference was -12.02 and 2.78 respectively while the Lowest difference was at 3D-LLM (-3.36 and 1.71 respectively)

Results are outlined in Table 6.

Groups		Retraction	Advancement
Measurements	N	Mean ± SD	Mean ± SD
3D-NL	20	-5.32 ± 8.11	3.82 ± 9.55
3D-Ph	20	-12.02 ± 0.86	2.78 ± 10.82
3D-LLM	20	-3.36 ± 1.16	1.71 ± 11.09

Table 6. Means and standard deviation for the percentage volume deformation at the facial folds on the soft tissue profile (%).

5. Correlation between two-dimensional and three-dimensional measurements

Current orthodontic research reports linear 2D or volumetric 3D changes in the facial soft tissues without establishing a relationship between 2D and 3D measurements. Knowing this relationship could enable clinicians to use 2D measurements as a routine tool to determine the behavior of the soft tissue of the face in the three planes of space. This can serve as a useful guide in diagnosis, treatment planning/ prediction and patient communication.

In an attempt to study the relationship between 3D morphologic measurements of soft tissue change following orthodontic treatment and the corresponding two-dimensional change, we (Al-Sanea, Kusnoto and Evans) tested the hypothesis that there is significant correlation between 3D morphologic measurements and 2D morphologic measurements of facial soft tissue change following orthodontic treatment in the same regions of the face in the same patient.

5.1 Correlation measurements between two-dimensional and three-dimensional changes in the soft tissue profile retraction group

Pearson correlation coefficient was calculated to determine the relationship between two-dimensional and three-dimensional measurements in the soft tissue profile retraction group at (0.05) level of significance. No statistically significant correlation existed between two-dimensional and three-dimensional measurements. The p values of the correlation ranged between (0.084- 0.661). Table 7 shows the Pearson Correlation values while scatter diagrams are represented in Figure 11-15.

Measurements	Number	ρ	Significance
2D-Sn and 3D- Sn	20	-0.173	NS
2D-SfA and 3D-SfA	20	0.212	NS
2D-UL and 3D-UL	20	-0.136	NS
2D-LL and 3D-LL	20	0.396	NS
2D-SfB and 3D-SfB	20	-0.104	NS

NS: Statistically non significant
*P value is statistically significant at 0.05

Table 7. Correlation measurements between two-dimensional and three dimensional changes in the soft tissue profile retraction group.

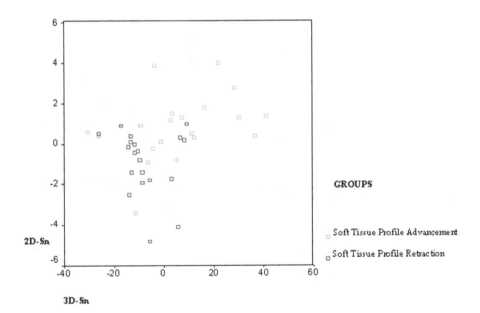

Fig. 11. Scatter diagram of correlation between 2D-Sn and 3D-Sn values.

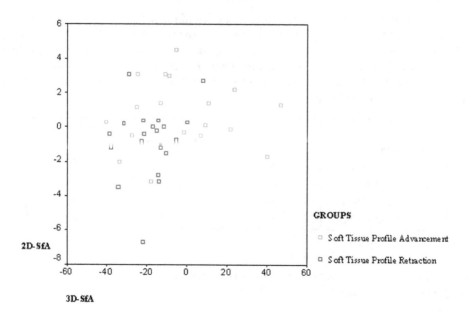

Fig. 12. Scatter diagram of correlation between 2D-SfA and 3D- SfA.

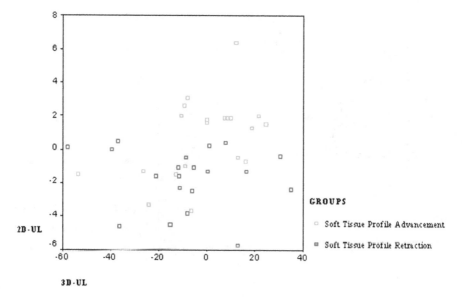

Fig. 13. Scatter diagram of correlation between 2D-UL and 3D- UL.

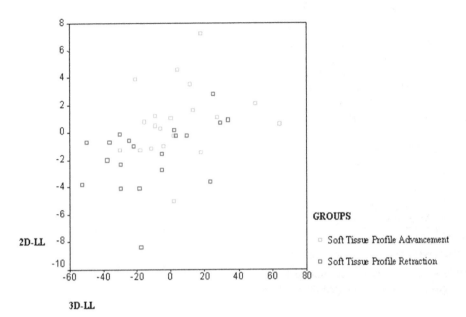

Fig. 14. Scatter diagram of correlation between 2D-LL and 3D-LL.

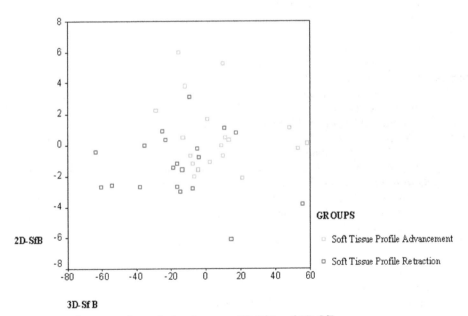

Fig. 15. Scatter diagram of correlation between 2D-SfB and 3D-SfB.

5.2 Correlation measurements between two-dimensional and three dimensional changes in the soft tissue profile advancement group

Pearson correlation coefficient was calculated to determine the relationship between two-dimensional and three-dimensional measurements in the soft tissue profile advancement group at (0.05) level of significance. No statistically significant correlation existed between two-dimensional and three-dimensional measurements except in the upper lip values (2D-UL and 3D-UL) where the p value was 0.033. The p values of the correlation in the rest of the measurements ranged between (0.116-0.917). The Pearson Correlation values and the scatter diagrams are shown in Table 8 and Figures 11-15 respectively.

Measurements	Number	p	Significance
2D-Sn and 3D- Sn	20	0.363	NS
2D-SfA and 3D-SfA	20	0.025	NS
2D-UL and 3D-UL	20	0.477*	S
2D-LL and 3D-LL	20	0.212	NS
2D-SfB and 3D-SfB	20	-0.207	NS

NS: Statistically non significant
*P value is statistically significant at 0.05

Table 8. Correlation measurements between two-dimensional and three dimensional changes in the soft tissue profile advancement group.

6. References

Al-Mesad, S. (1998). Soft Tissue Changes in White and Black Orthodontic Populations. Master's Thesis A447, University of Illinois at Chicago, Chicago, pp. 1-68.

Al-Sanea, R. (2007). Three Dimensional Morphometric Analysis of Facial Soft Tissue Changes Following Orthodontic Treatment. M.S. dissertation, University of Illinois at Chicago, United States – Illinois, Dissertations & Theses @ CIC Institutions, (Publication No. AAT 1449189), pp. 1-91, ISBN 9780549284208

Bishara, S.E.; Cummins, D.M. & Jakobsen, J.R. (1995). A Computer Assisted Photogrammetric Analysis of Soft Tissue Changes After Orthodontic Treatment, Part II: Results. *American Journal of Orthodontics and Dentofacial Orthopedics*, Vol.108, No.1, (July 1995), pp 38-47, ISSN 0889-5406

Blanz, V. & Vetter, T. (1999). A Morphable Model for the Synthesis of 3D Faces. *SIGGRAPH' 99 Conference Proceedings*, pp. 187-194, ISSN 0097-8930

Bloom, L.A. (1961). Perioral Profile Changes in Orthodontic Treatment. *American Journal of Orthodontics and Dentofacial Orthopedics*, 47:371, 1961, ISSN 0889-5406

Boley, J.C.; Pontier, J.P.; Smith, S. & Fulbright, M. (1998). Facial Changes in Extraction and Non-Extraction Patients. *Angle Orthodontist*, Vol.68, No.6, (December 1998), pp. 539-546, ISSN 0003-3219

Burke, P. (1983). Stereophotogrammetic Measurement of Change in Soft Tissue Following Surgery. *British Dental Journal*, Vol.155, No.11, (December 1983), pp. 373-379, ISSN 00007-0610

Clement, J.G. & Marks, M.K., eds. (2005) Computer-Graphic Facial Reconstruction . Amsterdam and Boston, Elsevier Academic Press, 2005, pp. 1-390, ISBN 0124730515

DeCarlo, D.; Metaxas, D. & Stone, M. (1998). An Anthropometric Face Model Using Variational Techniques. *SIGGRAPH' 98 Conference Proceedings*, pp. 67-74, ISSN 0097-8930

Denis, K.L. & Speidel, T.M. (1987). Comparison of the Three Methods of Profile Change Prediction in the Adult Orthodontic Patient. *American Journal of Orthodontics and Dentofacial Orthopedics*, Vol.92, No.5, (November 1987), pp. 376-402, ISSN 0889-5406

Farkas, L.G: (1987). Anthropometric Facial Proportions. Springfield, Charles C. Thomas Publisher, ISBN 0398052611

FaceGen™. (2005, 2009) Singular Inversions © 2005, 2009. Vancouver, British Columbia, Canada.

Finnoy, J.P.; Wisth, P.J. & Boe, O.E. (1987). Changes in Soft Tissue Profile During and After Orthodontic Treatment. *European Journal of Orthodontics*, Vol.9, No.1, (February 1987), pp. 68- 78, ISSN 0141-5387

Garner, L.D. (1974). Soft Tissue Changes Concurrent With Orthodontic Tooth Movement. *American Journal of Orthodontics and Dentofacial Orthopedics*, Vol.66, No.4, (October 1974), pp. 357–377, ISSN 0889-5406

Harrell, W.; Hatcher, D. & Bolt, R. (2002). In Search of Anatomic Truth: 3D Digital Patient Modeling and the Future of Orthodontics, *American Journal of Orthodontics and Dentofacial Orthopedics*, Vol.122, No.3, (September 2002), pp. 125-130, ISSN 0889-5406

Hatcher, D.C. & Dial, C. (1999). Dental Imaging Centers. *Journal of the California Dental Association*, Vol.27, No.12, (December 1999), pp. 953-9, ISSN 1043-2256

Hershey, H.G. (1972). Incisor Tooth Retraction and Subsequent Profile Change in Postadolescent Female Patients. *American Journal of Orthodontics and Dentofacial Orthopedics*, Vol.61, No.1, (January 1972), pp. 45–54, ISSN 0889-5406

Hutton, T.J.; Buxton, B.F.; Hammond, P. & Potts, H.W.W. (2003). IEEE Transactions on Medical Imaging. 22, 2003.

Ismail, S.F. & Moss, J.P. (2002). The Three-Dimensional Effects of Orthodontic Treatment on the Facial Soft Tissues - a Preliminary Study. *British Dental Journal*, Vol.192, No.2, (January 2002), pp. 104-108, ISSN 0007-0610

Kocadereli, I. (2002). Changes in Soft Tissue Profile After Orthodontic Treatment With and Without Extractions. *American Journal of Orthodontics and Dentofacial Orthopedics*, Vol.122. No.1, (July 2002), pp. 67-72, ISSN 0889-5406.

Lavelle, C.L., Carvalho, R.S.: An Evaluation of the Changes in Soft-Tissue Profile Form Induced by Orthodontic Therapy. *American Journal of Orthodontics and Dentofacial Orthopedics*, Vol.96, No.6, (December, 1989), pp. 467-476, ISSN 0889-5406

Lele, S. & Richtsmeire, J.T. (1991). Euclidean Distance Matrix Analysis: a Coordinate-Free Approach for Comparing Biological Shapes Using Landmark Data. *American Journal of Physical Anthropology*, Vol.86, No.3, (November 1991), pp. 415-427, ISSN 0002-9483

Lele, S. & Cole, T.M. (1995). Euclidean Distance Matrix Analysis: a Statistical Review. In: Current Issues in Statistical Shape Analysis, Eds. Mardia, K.K.V. & Gill, C.A., Leeds University Press, pp. 49-53, ISBN 0853161615

Luppanapornlarp, S. & Johnston, L.E. Jr. (1993). The Effects of Premolar-Extraction: a Long-Term Comparison of Outcomes in "Clear-Cut" Extraction and Nonextraction Class II Patients. *Angle Orthodontist*, Vol.64, No.4, (Winter 1993), pp. 257-272, ISSN 0003-3219

Marsh, J.L. & Vannier, M.V. (1983). The "Third Dimension" in Craniofacial Surgery. *Plastic and Reconstructive Surgery*, Vol.71, No.6, (June 1983), pp. 759-767, ISSN 0032-1052

Moss, J.P.; Linney, A.D.; Grindrod, S.R.; Ridge, S.R. & Clifton, J.S. (1987). Three-Dimensional Visualization of the Face and Skull Using Computerized Tomography and Laser Scaling Techniques. *American Journal of Orthodontics and Dentofacial Orthopedics*, Vol.94, No.4, (November 1987), pp. 247-253, ISSN 0089-5406

Moss, J.P. & Linney, A.D. (1990). The Prediction of Facial Aesthetics. *The New York State Dental Journal*, Vol.56, No.6, (June-July 1990), pp. 44-46, ISSN 0028-7571

Oliver, B.M. (1982). The Influence of Lip Thickness and Strain on Upper Lip Response to Incisor Retraction. *American Journal of Orthodontics and Dentofacial Orthopedics*, Vo.82, No.2, (August 1982), pp. 141-148, ISSN 0889-5406

O'Toole, A.J.; Vetter, T. & Blanz, V. (1999). Three-Dimensional Shape and Two-Dimensional Surface Reflectance Contributions to Face Recognition: An Application of Three-Dimensional Morphing. *Vision Research*, Vol.39, No.18, (September 1999), pp. 3145-3155, ISSN 0042-6989

Paquette, D.E.; Beattie, J.R. & Johnston, L.E. Jr. (1992). A Long-Term Comparison of Nonextraction and Premolar Extraction Edgewise Therapy in "Borderline" Class II Oatients. *American Journal of Orthodontics and Dentofacial Orthopedics*, Vol.102, No.1, (July 1992), pp. 1-14, ISSN 0889-5406

Peck, S. & Peck, L. (1995). Selected Aspects of the Art and Science of Facial Esthetics. *Seminars in Orthodontics*, Vol.1, No.1, (June 1995) pp. 105-126, ISSN 1073-8746

Quintero, J.C.; Trosien, A.; Hatcher D. & Kapila S. (1999). Craniofacial Imaging in Orthodontics: Historical Perspective, Current Status, and Future Developments. *Angle Orthodontist*, Vol.69, No.6, (December 1999), pp. 491-506, ISSN 0003-3219

Riedel, R.A. (1950). Esthetics and Its Relation to Orthodontic Therapy. *Angle Orthodontist*, Vol.20, No.3, (July 1950), pp. 168-78, ISSN 0003-3219

Roos, N. (1977). Soft Tissue Changes in Class II Treatment. *American Journal of Orthodontics and Dentofacial Orthopedics*, Vol.72, No.2, (August 1977), pp. 165-175, ISSN 0889-5406

Rudee, D.A. (1964). Proportional Profile Changes Concurrent With Orthodontic Therapy. *American Journal of Orthodontics and Dentofacial Orthopedics*, Vol.50, No.6, (June 1964), pp. 421-434, ISSN 0889-5406

Savara, B.S. (1965). Applications of Photogrammetry for Quantitative Study of Tooth and Face Morphology. *American Journal of Physical Anthropology*, Vol.23, No.4, (December 1965), pp. 427-434, ISSN 0002-9483

Singh, G.D.; Maldonado, L. & Thind, B.S. (2004-2005). Changes in the Soft Tissue Facial Profile Following Orthodontic Extractions: a Geometric Morphometric Study. *The Functional Orthodontist*, Vol.22, No.1, (Winter 2004-Spring 2005), pp. 34-38, 40, ISSN 8756-3150

Tweed, C. H. (1944). Indications for the Extraction of Teeth in Orthodontic Procedure. *American Journal of Orthodontics and Oral Surgery*, Vol.30, No.8, (August 1944), pp. 405-428, ISSN 0096-6347

Weisstein, E.W. (1999). Distance. From: *MathWorld--A Wolfram Web Resource*. http://mathworld.wolfram.com/Distance.html, 1999.

Wisth, P.J. (1974). Soft Tissue Response to Upper Incisor Retraction in Boys. *British Journal of Orthodontics*, Vol.1, No.5, (October 1974), pp. 199-204, ISSN 0301-228X

5

Other Applications of Photo Catalyst in Dental Treatments in Diverse Fields

Seung-Ho Ohk[1] and Hyeon-Shik Hwang[2]
[1]Department of Oral Microbiology,
[2]Department of Orthodontics and Dental Science
Research Institute, Chonnam National University
Korea

1. Introduction

Photocatalysts do not make the light faster. The term 'photocatalyst' represents chemical substances that act as a catalyst when exposed to light. For several decades numerous studies have been published about photocatalyst in water treatment process and air pollution control. Among several photocatalysts, TiO_2 has been considered as the most useful and harmless substance. With the illumination of UV-A light, TiO_2 photocatalysts decompose organic compounds through oxidation, with hydroxyl radicals ($HO\cdot$) being produced by the oxidation of water. Various methods have been introduced for the surface modification of orthodontic treatment devices. Among them, Sol-gel dip-coating, CVD and PE-CVD methods were applied to coat photocatalytic TiO_2 on the surface of orthodontic wires and brackets. The antibacterial activities of the surface-modified orthodontic wires and brackets were demonstrated on *Streptococcus mutans* and *Porphyromonas gingivalis*. Viable cell counts with dilution-agar plate method and spectrophotometry were carried out to evaluate the antibacterial effect of photocatalytic TiO_2. Besides the photocatalytic degradation of organic compounds, there are several unique characteristics of photocatalytic TiO_2 were reported. In virtue of those characteristics it can be used in various ways such as preventing air contamination, anti-fog glasses and anti-bacterial paints. Sometimes many useful points are considered as handicaps in other point of view and vice versa. For example, to show photocatalytic activity for the TiO_2, usually it needs illumination with wavelength of less than 380. However, this drawback could be, in turn, used as a useful tool to control the release of hydroxyl radical from water since there is not much of UV-A in normal sun light.

The definition of photocatalysts and basic mechanism of photocatalytic activity will be described in this chapter.

Application and evaluation methods of photocatalyst, antibacterial efficiency on oral pathogens and safety of photocatalyst will be mentioned also. With the advantage of photocatalytic TiO_2, safety, versatile applications and other important remarkable characteristics of photocatalytic TiO_2 will be described in this section.

2. What is photocatalyst?

2.1 Photochemical reaction

Does the 'photocatalyst' catalyze photo-reaction or catalyze reactions with the exposure of light? Literally, both of the meanings are correct. However, the later will be explained in this chapter.The term 'photocatalyst' represents chemical substance that act as a catalyst when exposed to light. 'Photocatalytic reaction' again can be classified as one of photo-reactions. The most popular example of photo-reaction is a photographic film. Although digital imaging technique is popular these days, one of the most excellent inventions was the development of photography. In a traditional way of taking photo, a target image was exposed to a roll of film installed in the dark space of camera. This photographic film is a sheet of plastic paper such as polyester, nitrocellulose or cellulose acetate coated with a light-sensitive silver bromide emulsion. When the emulsion is exposed to sufficient light, bromide ion (Br-) produces brom-atom and electron (e-). This electron, in turns, binds to silver ion (Ag+) to make metallic silver, which blocks light and appears as the black part of film negative.

$$Br^- + [light] \rightarrow Br + e^-$$

$$Ag^+ + e^- \rightarrow Ag$$

In 1972, Honda and Fujishima have reported electrochemical decomposition of water (Fujishima & Honda, 1972). They have found that when platinum and titanium dioxide (TiO_2) were connected as cathode and anode, respectively, water is decomposed with a illumination of xenon lamp to make hydrogen and oxygen molecules (Fig.1).

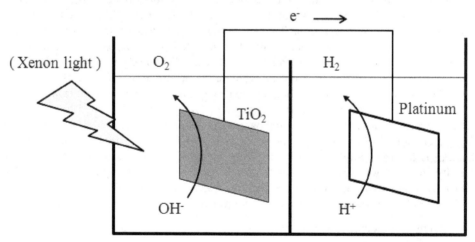

Fig. 1. Decomposition of water with photocatalytic TiO_2.

$$2H_2O + [Light, < 400 \text{ nm}] + TiO_2 \rightarrow 2H + O_2$$

This is a coupled reaction of reduction ($4H^+ \rightarrow 2H_2$) and oxidation ($4OH^- \rightarrow O_2 + 2H_2O$) with four molecules of water ($4H_2O$, $4H^+ + 4OH^-$) producing hydrogen and oxygen molecules.

Titanium dioxide can absorb light energy of below 400 nm and emits electrons to catalyze the decomposition of water.

2.2 Photocatalytic TiO$_2$

Several substances have been known to have photocatalytic activities such as ZnO, Nb$_2$O$_5$, WO$_3$, SnO$_2$, ZrO$_2$, CdS, ZnS, CdSe, and GaP. One of the most important reason that titanium dioxide is widely used is that it is chemically stable in most of acid, base and organic solvents. In the contrary, ZnO has similar energy band and high photocatalytic activity. However, when it is illuminated with light in aqueous solution, it can be easily dissolved in water as a Zn$^+$ ion. It also can be easily melt with sulfuric acid or nitric acid. Therefore, ZnO cannot be used separately.

3. Surface modification of orthodontic treatment devices

3.1 Anodic oxidation

When metal or silicon plates are immersed in an appropriate electrolyte a fine and rigid thin oxidized film will form on the surfaces plates. Anodic oxidation of aluminum is commonly introduced for their (semi-) transparent, anti-corrosion characteristics. The film composed by anodic oxidation usually shows stable conductivity. Neutral or acidic electrolytes are commonly used for aluminum, but there are not many options for other metals. Several dental implants have used anodic oxidation method for the surface modification to enhance their bone integration efficiency (Schupbach *et al.*, 2005).

3.2 Sol-gel dip-coating method

Dip-coating method is the oldest and most commonly used technique in deposition of thin film. Jenaer Glaswerk Schott & Gen are the first who have filed a patent with dip-coating technique for silica film in 1939. Sol-gel coatings, on the other hand, are being studied and applied in a diverse way such as protective coatings, passivation layers, ferroelectrics, sensors and membranes. The sol-gel dip-coating method uses inorganic precursors in aqueous or organic solvents. Those precursors are hydrolyzed and condensed to form polymers. Solid substrates are usually taken out of coating bath vertically at a constant speed. While taken out of the bath, the substrate entrains the liquid. Along with the evaporation of the solvent, wedge shaped film is formed on the surface of substrate. A lot of researchers have used sol-gel dip-coating method to study the application of the photocatalytic TiO$_2$ (Dongare *et al.*, 2003; Lee *et al.*, 2004; Zainal *et al.*, 2005).

3.3 CVD (Chemical vapor deposition) and PE-CVD (Plasma enhanced-CVD) method

Chemical vapor deposition method is the most widely used technique in semiconductor industries. It can form thin films from different precursors onto a substrate. In a CVD technique, a substrate is exposed to multiple volatile precursors with an inert gaseous carrier at high temperature and pressure. Those volatile precursors react or decompose on the surface of desired substrates, which form a thin film. Since CVD is one of the most well studied, and set up techniques, it is good for mass production.

Plasma enhanced CVD (PE-CVD) is a more progressed and important technique in VLSI (Very-large-scale integration) and TFT (Thin film transistor) manufacturing. The most important advantage of PE-CVD is low process temperature, which enables lower the manufacturer's budget. It uses plasma energy instead of heat energy for the reaction between precursors and substrates. Due to the wide range of applications of photocatalytic TiO$_2$, much of studies have been reported with CVD and PE-CVD technique for the application (Giavaresi et al., 2003; Gluszek et al., 1997; Gonzalez-Elipe et al., 2004; Mills et al., 2002).

4. Antibiotic effect of photocatalytic TiO$_2$

After Fujishima and Honda (Fujishima & Honda, 1972) reported the photolytic effect of TiO$_2$ in 1972, a series of efforts have been carried out to apply in various ways. Among them Matsunaga et al. have first reported photocatalytic TiO$_2$ has antibacterial effect on *Lactobacillus acidophilus*, *Saccharomyces cerevisiae* and *Escherichia coli* (Matsunaga et al., 1985). Since hydroxyl radical (HO•) became of interest in decomposing organic compounds, it is no wonder to try antibacterial effect on various microorganisms. It was well documented that chemical oxidation with hydroxyl radical has a high activity in degradation of organic compounds (Ireland & Valinieks, 1992). Accordingly, antibacterial effect of photocatalytic TiO$_2$ that could efficiently produce hydroxyl radical in aqueous solution with illumination of light was demonstrated. Major microorganisms that have tested with photocatalytic TiO$_2$ were listed in Table 1.

According to the early report presented by Ireland et al. *Escherichia coli* showed rapid cell death in a mixture with the anatase crystalline form of titanium dioxide (Ireland et al., 1993). Cho et al. also explained correlation between HO• radicals and the rate of *E. coli* inactivation which indicates that the HO• radical is the primary oxidant species responsible for inactivating *E. coli* in the UV/TiO$_2$ process (Cho et al., 2004). Effort to clarify the antibacterial effect of titanium plate by surface modifications has been also reported. Yoshinari et al. tried to modify the surface of titanium plate by ion implantation (Ca$^+$, N$^+$, and F$^+$), oxidation (anode oxidation, titania spraying), ion plating (TiN, alumina), and ion beam mixing (Ag, Sn, Zn, Pt) with Ar$^+$ (Yoshinari et al., 2001). Among them they have reported that F$^+$-implanted specimens significantly inhibited the growth of both *Porphyromonas gingivalis* and *Actinobacillus actinomycetemcomitans*. However, this antibacterial effect might be caused by the formation of a metal fluoride complex on the surfaces.

Since orthodontic wires and brackets provide a sufficient habitat for oral infectious microorganisms, orthodontic patients might have a higher risk of contracting other dental diseases (Balenseifen & Madonia, 1970; Sakamaki & Bahn, 1968; Scheie et al., 1984). Therefore, as well as the orthodontic patients, clinicians should pay attention to reduce the chances for oral microorganisms to adhere to the surfaces of teeth and orthodontic wires. Chun et al. have tried to apply photocatalytic TiO$_2$ to orthodontic wires (Chun et al., 2007). They used sol-gel dip coating method to modify the surfaces of wires. Special device for efficient illumination of UV-light to TiO$_2$-coated orthodontic wires using quartz cylinder was designed and used for the adhesion assay (Fig. 2). Since *Streptococcus mutans* that causes dental caries can easily adhere to tooth surface or orthodontic devices attached to tooth surfaces anti-adhesion effect of photocatalytic TiO$_2$ was monitored. Modified surface of wires showed effectively reduced adhesion of bacterial cells. Surface modification with photocatalytic TiO_2 enabled orthodontic wires to have effective anti-adherent characteristics. Using Scanning electron microscope damaged bacterial cell surfaces could be observed when treated with TiO_2. Similar effect was observed in *Porphyromonas gingivalis*, which is known as one of the major pathogen of periodontitis.

	Species	References
Bacteria	*Escherichia coli*	(Cho *et al.*, 2004; Ireland *et al.*, 1993; Kuhn *et al.*, 2003; Matsunaga *et al.*, 1985; Salih, 2002)
	Lactobacillus acidophilus	(Matsunaga *et al.*, 1985)
	Saccharomyces cerevisiae	(Matsunaga *et al.*, 1985)
	Streptococcus mutans	(Chun *et al.*, 2007; Elsaka *et al.*, 2011)
	Porphyromonas gingivalis	(Chun *et al.*, 2007; Yoshinari *et al.*, 2001)
	Bacillus atrophaeus	(Muranyi *et al.*, 2010)
	Kocuria rhizophila	(Muranyi *et al.*, 2010)
	Pseudomonas aeruginosa	(Kuhn *et al.*, 2003)
	Staphylococcus aureus	(Kuhn *et al.*, 2003)
	Enterococcus faecium	(Kuhn *et al.*, 2003)
Fungi	*Aspergillus niger*	(Muranyi *et al.*, 2010)
Yeast	*Candida albicans*	(Kuhn *et al.*, 2003)
Viruses	Rota virus	(Sang *et al.*, 2007)
	Astrovirus	(Sang *et al.*, 2007)
	Feline calcivirus (FCV)	(Sang *et al.*, 2007)
	Bacteriophage	(Gerrity *et al.*, 2008; Liga *et al.*, 2011)
Prion	PrP[SC]	(Paspaltsis *et al.*, 2006)

Table 1. Major microorganisms that have positive results with photocatalytic TiO_2.

Other than antibacterial effect, the efficacies of TiO_2 on viruses and prion have also demonstrated. Sang *et al.* have tested rotavirus, astrovirus, and feline calcivirus (FCV) to verify the inactivation effect of TiO_2 with irradiation of visible light (Sang *et al.*, 2007). According to the report, light activated TiO_2 could partially degrade dsRNA of the rotavirus particles. They have found that activated TiO_2 with illumination of light in aqueous solution produces a significant amount of reactive oxygen species such as superoxide anions (O_2^-) and hydroxyl radicals ($\bullet OH$) after activation for 8, 16, and 24 hrs. Destruction of nucleic acid was also confirmed by Ashikaga *et al.* (Ashikaga *et al.*, 2000). Those reactive oxygen species affect not only nucleotides but also other organic compounds such as peptides or proteins. With this special features, Paspaltsis *et al.* have examined the photocatalytic TiO_2 to prion protein, which is known to cause transmissible spongiform encephalopathy (TSB) (Paspaltsis *et al.*, 2006). Inoculation of prion protein (PrP[SC]) with a TiO_2/H_2O_2 treatment to Syrian hamsters showed higher survival rate than control group and retarded presentation of clinical symptom for 50 days later. Since prion is strongly resistant to commonly used conventional decontamination methods, they have presented photocatalytic TiO$_2$ as a potential disinfecting agent for liquid waste and TSE infectious agent.

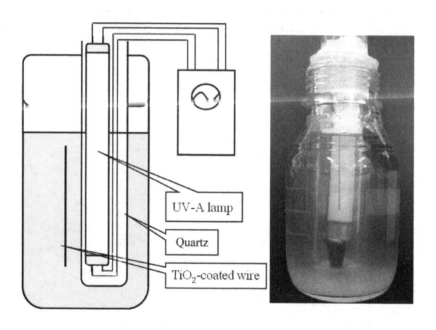

Fig. 2. Apparatus for the assay of anti-adhesion effect of TiO$_2$-coated orthodontic wire.

5. Other applications of photo catalyst in dental treatments

We are unconsciously in contact with diverse form of titanium dioxide these days. It is now commonly used in making papers, fabrics, toothpastes and wall paints. Photocatalytic TiO$_2$ has a broad spectrum of applications in virtue of its almighty capability of degrading almost every organic compounds. It has been realized that TiO$_2$ can absorb energy from light (usually UV light) and react with water molecules to produce reactive oxygen species.

One of the main focuses of applying photocatalytic TiO$_2$ was decontamination of polluted environments such as air cleaning system, decomposition of waste water. At the beginning of studies on the photocatalytic TiO$_2$, it was mainly applied to degrade highly toxic dyes from textile industries (Muneer et al., 1997; Saquib & Muneer, 2003). However, its scope has been gradually expanded to various areas such as herbicides (Singh et al., 2003) or pesticides (Daneshvar et al., 2004) and other industrial waste water (Makino et al., 2007).

Several companies producing ceramic tiles are using TiO$_2$ on the very surface of their products which is so-called self-cleaning tiles. Due to the ability to decompose organic molecules, these self-cleaning tiles can disinfect contamination of their surfaces by themselves only if there's a little portion of moisture and enough sun light. It might be very useful in hospitals, public restrooms, and household bathrooms. This unique advantage can be expanded to trivial devices used in most of clinics such as forceps, spatulas, scissors, and any rigid ceramic or metal surfaces to reduce the opportunity of cross infection.

Another useful aspect of TiO_2 is the hydrophilic property. Coating with photocatalytic TiO_2 layer on rigid ceramic or metal surfaces provides super-hydrophilic property that might dramatically reduce contact angle. Ohdaira *et al.* in Department of General Surgery, Jichi Medical Universitym Japan have designed special laparoscope that has antifogging effect (Ohdaira *et al.*, 2007). This property also can be applied to dental mirrors, bathroom mirrors, and car windows to impose antifogging characteristics.

6. Limitations and drawbacks of photocatalytic TiO_2

Even though photocatalytic TiO_2 has various utilities and potentials, still it has some limitations and drawbacks. It still needs improvements in reaction rate, broad spectrum of light source, specificity (or wide range of target) and stability. Several limitations and expected solutions are listed in Table 2. However, many of these are not solved yet.

Limitations	Solutions
Low reaction rate	Increasing surface area
Incomplete reaction	Fluid type reactor
Low efficiency	Increasing surface area
	Gas type reactor
Low specificity	Reactor design for specifically adsorption of target substances
Light source	Mixing with other inorganic compounds

Table 2. Several limitations of photocatalytic TiO_2.

6.1 Surface area

Since photocatalytic reaction occurs at the solid surface of TiO_2, it is very easy to separate substrates or products from photocatalyst. However substrates should be in contact with photocatalyst, which causes relatively low reaction rate and less homogeneity compared to other reactions such as gas-gas, or liquid-gas reactions. The first way to manage this problem is to increase surface area of the catalysts and the way to increase surface area is to reduce the particle sizes. Some solid catalysts are used in a unique three dimensional structure such as 'honey comb structure' to increase surface area. However it is not suitable for the photocatalytic TiO_2 because it needs illumination of UV or day light to activate. Therefore making round shaped particles and reduction in size may be the only way to increase surface area. Average diameter of commonly used TiO_2 ranges from 20 nm to 0.5 μm. Ultrafine particles of even below 10 nm of diameter are now developed and used in some fields. The average surface area of some ultrafine particle is reduced down to 7 nm which has about 300 m^2/g of surface area. Photocatalytic activity of this particle is 2 – 4 times higher than the particle that has 50 m^2/g of surface area. The activity did not increase as much as the surface area because ultrafine particles usually can aggregate each other. But there is no reason not to use ultrafine particles if it shows higher activity even though increasing fold of activity is not high as that of surface area.

6.2 Crystalline forms

Titanium dioxide forms three kinds of crystals: those are rutile, anatase, and brookite (Fig. 3). It is usually said that anatase crystal has higher photocatalytic activity than others. Depending on the crystalline type, binding structure of T-O and characteristics of crystal surface varies of course. However, the reason is unclear until now. Anatase crystal of TiO_2 can be formed between 400 – 500 °C and transformed to rutile at more than 900 °C.

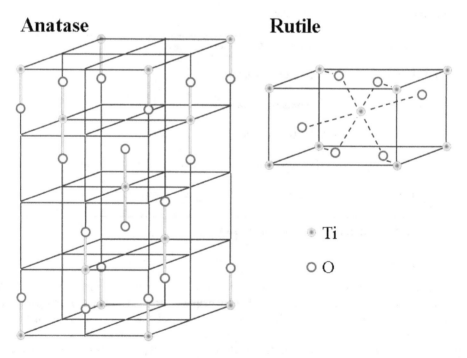

Fig. 3. Anatase and rutile forms of crystalline TiO_2.

6.3 Light sources

As the term 'photo-' represents, illumination of light is essential for the photocatalytic TiO_2 to get catalytic activity. It is the most important limitation in designing reactors with photocatalytic TiO_2. Even worse is the fact that most of photocatalytic TiO_2 can only utilize UV rather than visible light. It may not be a drawback of TiO_2, if any devices or reactors use natural sun light as a light source. However, in the view point of energy efficiency, if the reactor can utilize only a part of natural sun light and cannot utilize visible light, energy efficiency of the reactor will be less than 5% at most. Some of physical or chemical changes of titanium dioxide should be necessary to absorb and utilize visible light. Otherwise, photocatalytic TiO_2 can utilize visible light by mixing a small amount of other inorganic substances such as chromic oxide (Cr_2O_3, VI). However, in this case, reduced photocatalytic activity should be expected.

Limitation of light source may not always be a drawback of photocatalytic TiO_2. Since it produces hydroxyl radicals in aqueous solution and hydroxyl radical can decompose most of organic compounds, prolonged release of hydroxyl radical might be harmful in living organisms such as human. In case of antibacterial orthodontic wire described in section 3, it was coated with photocatalytic TiO_2 for its additional feature. The fact that releases of hydroxyl radicals from the photocatalytic TiO_2 for decomposition of bacterial cell wall compartments may imply a negative supposition. Hydroxyl radicals may also act on normal oral epithelial cells. In this case, the limitation of TiO_2 could, in turn, be a simple solution for the problem. The fact that relatively low intensity of UV light in normal day light is an advantage in this case. Since, photocatalytic activity of TiO_2 is usually activated by UV light, it can be regulated by manually controlling the illumination time and period in dental clinics.

7. Conclusion

When Fujishima and Honda reported the remarkable characteristics of titanium dioxide in 1972, few people have noticed the potentials of this white powder. Combined with the powerful effect of reactive oxygen species it became an almost almighty substance that can be used in environmental cleanup industries, personal hygiene products and even food industries. Not many substances have been interested in such diverse fields. However, there are still some drawbacks to overcome in the application of photocatalytic TiO_2. That means it is still worthy of challenge in the field of photocatalysis research.

8. References

Ashikaga, T., Wada, M., Kobayashi, H., Mori, M., Katsumura, Y., Fukui, H., Kato, S., Yamaguchi, M. & Takamatsu, T. (2000) Effect of the photocatalytic activity of TiO_2 on plasmid DNA. *Mutation research*, 466, 1-7.

Balenseifen, J. W. & Madonia, J. V. (1970) Study of dental plaque in orthodontic patients. *Journal of dental research*, 49, 320-324.

Cho, M., Chung, H., Choi, W. & Yoon, J. (2004) Linear correlation between inactivation of E. coli and OH radical concentration in TiO_2 photocatalytic disinfection. *Water research*, 38, 1069-1077.

Chun, M. J., Shim, E., Kho, E. H., Park, K. J., Jung, J., Kim, J. M., Kim, B., Lee, K. H., Cho, D. L., Bai, D. H., Lee, S. I., Hwang, H. S., and Ohk, S. H. (2007) Surface modification of orthodontic wires with photocatalytic titanium oxide for its antiadherent and antibacterial properties. *The Angle orthodontist*, 77, 483-488.

Daneshvar, N., Hejazi, M. J., Rangarangy, B. & Khataee, A. R. (2004) Photocatalytic degradation of an organophosphorus pesticide phosalone in aqueous suspensions of titanium dioxide. *Journal of environmental science and health Part B, Pesticides, food contaminants, and agricultural wastes*, 39, 285-296.

Dongare, M. K., Sonawane, R. S. & Hegde, S. G. (2003) Preparation of titanium(IV) oxide thin film photocatalyst by sol-gel dip coating. *Mater Chem Phys*, 77, 744-750.

Elsaka, S. E., Hamouda, I. M. & Swain, M. V. (2011) Titanium dioxide nanoparticles addition to a conventional glass ionomer restorative. Influence on physical and antibacterial properties. *Journal of dentistry*, 39, 589-598.

Fujishima, A. & Honda, K. (1972) Electrochemical photolysis of water at a semiconductor electrode. *Nature*, 238, 37-38.

Gerrity, D., Ryu, H., Crittenden, J. & Abbaszadegan, M. (2008) Photocatalytic inactivation of viruses using titanium dioxide nanoparticles and low-pressure UV light. *Journal of environmental science and health Part A, Toxic/hazardous substances & environmental engineering*, 43, 1261-1270.

Giavaresi, G., Giardino, R., Ambrosio, L., Battiston, G., Gerbasi, R., Fini, M., Rimondini, L. & Torricelli, P. (2003) In vitro biocompatibility of titanium oxide for prosthetic devices nanostructured by low pressure metal-organic chemical vapor deposition. *The International journal of artificial organs*, 26, 774-780.

Gluszek, J., Masalski, J., Furman, P. & Nitsch, K. (1997) Structural and electrochemical examinations of PACVD TiO_2 films in Ringer solution. *Biomaterials*, 18, 789-794.

Gonzalez-Elipe, A. R., Gracia, F. & Holgado, J. P. (2004) Photoefficiency and optical, microstructural, and structural properties of TiO_2 thin films used as photoanodes. *Langmuir*, 20, 1688-1697.

Ireland, J. C. & Valinieks, J. (1992) Rapid measurement of aqueous hydroxyl radical concentrations in steady-state HO · flux systems. *Chemosphere*, 25, 383-396.

Ireland, J. C., Klostermann, P., Rice, E. W. & Clark, R. M. (1993) Inactivation of *Escherichia coli* by titanium dioxide photocatalytic oxidation. *Applied and environmental microbiology*, 59, 1668-1670.

Kuhn, K. P., Chaberny, I. F., Massholder, K., Stickler, M., Benz, V. W., Sonntag, H. G. & Erdinger, L. (2003) Disinfection of surfaces by photocatalytic oxidation with titanium dioxide and UVA light. *Chemosphere*, 53, 71-77.

Lee, J. M., Kim, M. S. & Kim, B. W. (2004) Photodegradation of bisphenol-A with TiO_2 immobilized on the glass tubes including the UV light lamps. *Water research*, 38, 3605-3613.

Liga, M. V., Bryant, E. L., Colvin, V. L. & Li, Q. (2011) Virus inactivation by silver doped titanium dioxide nanoparticles for drinking water treatment. *Water research*, 45, 535-544.

Makino, T., Matsumoto, K., Ebara, T., Mine, T., Ohtsuka, T. & Mizuguchi, J. (2007) Complete decomposition of benzene, toluene, and particulate matter contained in the exhaust of diesel engines by means of thermally excited holes in titanium dioxide at high temperatures. *Jpn J Appl Phys 1*, 46, 6037-6042.

Matsunaga, T., Tomoda, R., Nakajima, T. & Wakea, H. (1985) Photoelectrochemical sterilization of microbial cells by semiconductor powders. *FEMS Microbiology Letters*, 29, 211-214.

Mills, A., Lee, S. K., Lepre, A., Parkin, I. P. & O'Neill, S. A. (2002) Spectral and photocatalytic characteristics of TiO$_2$ CVD films on quartz. *Photochemical & photobiological sciences : Official journal of the European Photochemistry Association and the European Society for Photobiology*, 1, 865-868.

Muneer, M., Philip, R. & Das, S. (1997) Photocatalytic degradation of waste water pollutants. Titanium dioxide-mediated oxidation of a textile dye, acid blue 40. *Res Chem Intermediat*, 23, 233-246.

Muranyi, P., Schraml, C. & Wunderlich, J. (2010) Antimicrobial efficiency of titanium dioxide-coated surfaces. *Journal of applied microbiology*, 108, 1966-1973.

Ohdaira, T., Nagai, H., Kayano, S. & Kazuhito, H. (2007) Antifogging effects of a socket-type device with the superhydrophilic, titanium dioxide-coated glass for the laparoscope. *Surgical endoscopy*, 21, 333-338.

Paspaltsis, I., Kotta, K., Lagoudaki, R., Grigoriadis, N., Poulios, I. & Sklaviadis, T. (2006) Titanium dioxide photocatalytic inactivation of prions. *The Journal of general virology*, 87, 3125-3130.

Sakamaki, S. T. & Bahn, A. N. (1968) Effect of orthodontic banding on localized oral lactobacilli. *Journal of dental research*, 47, 275-279.

Salih, F. M. (2002) Enhancement of solar inactivation of *Escherichia coli* by titanium dioxide photocatalytic oxidation. *Journal of applied microbiology*, 92, 920-926.

Sang, X., Phan, T. G., Sugihara, S., Yagyu, F., Okitsu, S., Maneekarn, N., Muller, W. E. & Ushijima, H. (2007) Photocatalytic inactivation of diarrheal viruses by visible-light-catalytic titanium dioxide. *Clinical laboratory*, 53, 413-421.

Saquib, M. & Muneer, M. (2003) Photocatalytic degradation of two selected textile dye derivatives, eosine yellowish and p-rosaniline, in aqueous suspensions of titanium dioxide. *Journal of environmental science and health Part A, Toxic/hazardous substances & environmental engineering*, 38, 2581-2598.

Scheie, A. A., Arneberg, P. & Krogstad, O. (1984) Effect of orthodontic treatment on prevalence of *Streptococcus mutans* in plaque and saliva. *Scandinavian journal of dental research*, 92, 211-217.

Schupbach, P., Glauser, R., Rocci, A., Martignoni, M., Sennerby, L., Lundgren, A. & Gottlow, J. (2005) The human bone-oxidized titanium implant interface: A light microscopic, scanning electron microscopic, back-scatter scanning electron microscopic, and energy-dispersive x-ray study of clinically retrieved dental implants. *Clinical implant dentistry and related research*, 7 Suppl 1, S36-43.

Singh, H. K., Muneer, M. & Bahnemann, D. (2003) Photocatalysed degradation of a herbicide derivative, bromacil, in aqueous suspensions of titanium dioxide. *Photochemical & photobiological sciences : Official journal of the European Photochemistry Association and the European Society for Photobiology*, 2, 151-156.

Yoshinari, M., Oda, Y., Kato, T. & Okuda, K. (2001) Influence of surface modifications to titanium on antibacterial activity in vitro. *Biomaterials,* 22, 2043-2048.

Zainal, Z., Lee, C. Y., Hussein, M. Z., Kassim, A. & Yusof, N. A. (2005) Electrochemical-assisted photodegradation of dye on TiO_2 thin films: investigation on the effect of operational parameters. *Journal of hazardous materials,* 118, 197-203.

Part 2

Growth and Genetic

6

A Simplified Method to Determine the Potential Growth in Orthodontics Patients

Gladia Toledo Mayarí
School of Dentistry/ Havana Medical University
Cuba

1. Introduction

The current Orthodontics worries is about the early correction of malocclusion, giving importance to the harmonization of the bone bases in connection with the discrepancy and positioning of the teeth, that can be corrected in any time of life, for what is of great importance is to know the biggest peak of growth (Peluffo, 2001; Quirós 2000).

The maturation stages can have a considerable influence in the diagnosis, the goals of the treatment, the planning and the eventual result of the orthodontic treatment (Madhu et al., 2003; Toledo 2004).

The clinical decisions with regards to the use of the extraoral force, functional appliances, the treatment without extractions and the orthognatic surgeon is based on the considerations of the growth, for this reason, the prediction of the quantity of active growth, mainly in the craniofacial complex, are useful to the orthodontists (Toledo, 2004).

The orthodontic diagnosis has a group of stages in those that have multiple evaluation factors which are used in the study of the malocclusions. In general evaluation of a patient, it is important to consider the general physical development and the potential growth (Quirós 2000).

The pubertal growth spurt of is an advantageous period in the orthodontic treatment and it should be kept in mind in connection with the planning of the treatment. One of the objectives of the orthodontic treatment during the adolescence, in the cases with skeletal discrepancies is to take advantage of the changes of growth of the patient. (Fiani, 1998; Padrós & Creus, 2002).

In the adolescent, the phase of somatic maturity can influence in the selection of the appliances, the course of the treatment and the retention after the therapy (Geran et al. 2006). Because of this the study and the knowledge of the maturation stage and the phase of growth of the patient, is very important for making more efficient therapy. Authors like Nanda (Nanda, 1955), Björk and Helm (Björk & Helm, 1967), and Hägg and Taranger (Hägg & Taranger, 1980a, 1980b, 1982) established that the pattern of growth and facial development is similar to that of the general skeletal growth, and that the maximum peak of pubertal growth of the craniofacial structures occurs between 6 and 8 months after the maximum peak of pubertal growth in the stature.

Due to the wide individual variation, the chronological age cannot be used in the evaluation of the pubertal growth (Fiani, 1998), for that reason is appealed to determine the biological age. It is calculated starting from the bone, dental, morphological and sexual ages (Ceglia, 2005).

The study of the bone maturation is the surest and reliable method to evaluate the biological age of the individuals and to fix the physiologic maturity (Gutiérrez Muñiz et al. 2006).

In spite of the difficulties that outline the different existent methods (quality of the X-ray, minimum modifications of the projection, variability intra and inter observant, errors in the reading of the online systems, population in which the method is based, etc.) the evaluation of the bone maturation is indispensable in the clinical practice, since it is a parameter of great importance in the study of the alterations of the growth (Paesano et al, 1998).

The hand, the wrist and the distal epiphysis of the radius and the ulna present a great number of secondary centers of ossification on the whole, and they can reproduce in a single X-ray. For this reason, they are often chosen as study centers when it is sought to determine the state of skeletal maturation, although other centers of ossification of secondary epiphysis can be used, such as, the elbow and the tarsal bones (Cha, 2003).

Todd, in 1937, was the first author that mentioned the term "determinant of the maturity", when referring to the gradual changes that occur on the growth of the cartilage during the trial of coalition of the epiphysis with the diaphysis and that they can be determined by studying radiographic plaques (Quirós Álvarez, 2006). Years later Greulich and Pyle called them indicators of maturity and in 1959 they established the norms of skeletal age to value the bone maturation of the complete hand (Greulich & Pyle, 1959). As the different epiphyses don't often mature at the same time, discrepancies that are resolved with subjective trials which subtract precision to the method arise (Tanner et al. 1983).

Tanner and Whitehouse (Tanner et al. 1983), develop the method Tanner - Whitehouse 2 (TW2) to evaluate the bone development, through X-rays of the lefts hand and wrist, which has had great acceptance for their precision, being used at the present time in numerous countries (Izaguirre de Espinoza et al. 2003; Jiménez Hernández et al., 1986; Ortega et al., 2006).

In 1979, the professor Jordan (Jordan, 1979) publishes the results of the Study of Physical Growth in Cuba, where it uses the method TW2 in the determination of the bone maturation. Later on, in 1987 a group of investigators of the Department of Growth and Human Development determine the patterns of the Cuban population's bone maturation for sex and race through the method TW2 (Jiménez JM et al., 1987). This method is one of those that is used in Cuba in the evaluation of the bone maturation (Abreu Suárez et al., 1995).

Some authors have looked in the X-rays of the hand specific indicators of the spurt of pubertal growth (Fishman, 1982). Björk and Helm (Björk & Helm, 1967) and Gupta (Gupta, 1995) point out as a reliable indicator of the installation of the puberty, the beginning of the ossification of the sesamoid bone. Toledo (Toledo, 2004) and Rakosi and Jonas (Rakosi & Jonas, 1992) affirm that the appearance of the hook of the hamate bone is also a good indicator of the installation of the puberty.

In Maxillary Orthopedics one of the most utilized methods in the evaluation of the growth potential has been the one of Grave and Brown (Rakosi & Jonas, 1992; Tedaldi et al., 2007) that it divides the process of maturation of the bones of the hand in nine stages, between the 9th and the 17th year of age. The ossification characteristics are detected to the level of the phalanges, bones of the carpus and radius, and the stages of growth of the fingers are valued according to the relationship between the epiphysis and the diaphysis (Fiani, 1998). The evaluation of the Grave and Brown's method is recommended by Ortiz et al. (Ortiz et al., 2007), Spinelli Casanova et al. (Spinelli Casanova et al, 2006) and Pancherz and Hägg (Pancherz & Hägg, 1985) before the therapeutic interceptive in Orthodontics patients, to choose the ideal treatment according to the stages of bone maturation that the patient presents, diminishing this way the time in the use of the appliances and making them more effective. Previous to the realization of this investigation (Toledo Mayarí & Otaño Lugo, 2010a, 2010b, 2010c), was not reported in Cuba the use of Grave and Brown's method.

The inconvenience that presents the evaluation of the bone maturation through the hand in orthodontics patients , is the use of an additional X-ray for the patient, besides that this is not carried out with the dental X-ray machine, being necessary to remit the patient to a radiology service.

The current tendency in Orthodontics is to reduce the number of X-rays to the strictly necessary ones (Bujaldón Daza et al., 1998), for that indexes of skeletal maturation have been developed with the profiles of the bodies of the cervical vertebras that generally appear in the lateral teleradiography of skull used for the orthodontist diagnostic (Ortiz et al., 2007), being discharges correlations in the evaluations of the bone age between the cervical vertebras and the bones of the hand (Edilmar et al., 2005; Gandini et al., 2006; Hassel & Farman, 1995; San Roman et al., 2002; Uysal et al., 2006).

Also with the objective of substituting the X-ray of the hand that constitutes an additional exhibition to radiations in the patients of Orthodontics, Leite et al. (Leite et al., 1987), analyze the first three fingers, which include in the lateral teleradiography of skull and they don't find significant differences between the analysis of the bone maturation of the total hand and that of the three fingers. Shigemi Goto et al. (Shigemi Goto et al., 1996) and Rossi et al. (Rossi et al., 1999), analyze the changes at level of the first finger, in the distal phalanx and in the proximal respectively, finding that the evaluations at level of the phalanges constitute a quick and useful clinical method, to evaluate the growth potential in patient of Orthodontics. Madhu et al. (Madhu et al., 2003) and Ozer et al.((Ozer et al., 2006) use the stages of maturation of the middle phalange of the third finger, visualized in an X-ray of 41x31mm., taken with a machine of dental X rays conventional, where they find out that the evaluation of the stages of maturation of the middle phalanx of the third finger, constitutes an alternative method that can be used to determine the bone maturation, of the children in growth. Previous to the realization of this investigation, was not reports that in Cuba the patient's growth potential was evaluated through the middle phalange of the third finger, that which motivated us to determine the stages of maturation of that phalange and to identify the concordance between these and the stages of skeletal maturation, whereas clause that of existing concordance among the same ones, we will have a simplified method, for the determination of the growth potential, without the necessity of using an X-ray of the hand and an additional X-rays machine.

Problem of Investigation:

Whereas clause that in Orthodontics the evaluation of the growth potential has influence in the diagnosis, the treatment plan, the results and the prognostic of the treatment, and that the evaluation of the bone maturation through the X-ray of the hand, that is the anatomical area that is used in the evaluation of the bone maturation in Cuba, constitutes an additional X-ray for the tributary patients of orthodontist treatment, it would be necessary to respond:

What is the bone age of our patients?

What stages of skeletal maturation and of maturation of the middle phalange of the third finger they do present the same ones?

What is the relationship between the bone age and the chronological age, the stages of skeletal maturation and the stages of maturation of the middle phalange of the third finger in our patients?

What concordance does it exist among the methods to determine the growth potential in patient of Orthodontics?

The formulation of these questions forms the bases of a hypothesis that can be defined as it continues:

Considering that the growth potential constitutes the grade of growth becomes for the individual between the state in the moment of the exam and the definitive ceasing of this. In the determination of this potential, inside the diagnosis in Orthodontics, you can substitute the radiographic of the hand, being clinically useful the analysis of the bone maturation through the middle phalange of the third finger.

To give answers to the questions and the hypothesis, the following objectives were formulated:

General objective: To propose a simplified method to determine the growth potential in Orthodontics patient.

Specific objectives:

1. To determine according to sex and chronological age: the bone age, the stages of skeletal maturation and the stages of maturation of the middle phalange of the third finger.
2. To identify the relationship between the bone age and: the chronological age, the stages of skeletal maturation and the stages of maturation of the middle phalange of the third finger.
3. To identify the concordance between the studied methods.

2. Background

In this epigraph are approached theoretical aspects of great importance in the specialty of Orthodontics that were considered in this investigation, due to the great majority of the children that go to the clinic and they are tributary of orthodontic treatment, they are in periods of growth and development, reason why when ignoring their biological age, we could incur in errors when outlining a diagnosis, prognostic and treatment plan.

The terms of growth and development are used to indicate the series of changes of volume, forms and weight that suffers the organism from the fecundation until the mature age (Cannut Brusola, 1988; J. Mayoral & G. Mayoral, 1990).

The growth in an individual's active development, is a continuous phenomenon that begins in the moment of the conception and it culminates at the end of the puberty, period during which reaches the maturity in their physical, psycho-social and reproductive aspects. Both processes have characteristic communes to all the individuals of the same species, what makes them predictable, however, they present wide differences between the subjects, given by the pattern's of growth individual character and development. This typical pattern emerges on one hand of the interaction of genetic and environmental factors that establish the growth potential and for other, the magnitude that this potential is expressed (Proffit, 1994).

The chronological age, that constitutes the time lapsed from the birth until the moment of the exam (Proffit, 1994), it doesn't always allow to value the development and the patient's somatic maturation, for that is appear to determine the biological maturity (Fiani, 1998).

According to Gutiérrez Muñiz et al. (Gutiérrez Muñiz et al., 2006) "the concept of biological maturity is defined as the successive transformations through the time, from the conception until the adulthood, existing two applicable fundamental methods at the present time for its evaluation: the bone age and the dental age".

The bone age is established determining radiograph of the number and size of the centers of ossification epiphysis, which should be compared with the existent norms for each age and sex (Recalde Cortes et al. 1997; Tanner et al., 1983). Each bone begins with a primary center of ossification that will grow progressively at the same time that is remodeled being able to acquire an or more epiphysis and finally it will acquire the mature form with the coalition from the epiphysis to the body of the bone. The sequence for each bone is the same as for the events that will happen in it, taking place independently late to the grade or advance with regard to the chronological age (Cattani 2003; Fiani, 1998; Proffit, 1994).

The potential growth constitutes the grade of growth becomes for the individual between the state in the moment of the exam and the definitive ceasing of this (Proffit, 1994). It is given by the existent relationship between the bone age and the chronological age: to smaller bone age for a certain chronological age the individual's growth potential will be bigger, that is to say, the grade late of the bone age in connection with the chronological age reflects theoretically the years of growth residual extra or, that is the same thing, the years of growth that he has left before the closing of the epiphysis (Cattani 2003; Proffit, 1994).

Theoretically, any part of the body can be used to determine the bone age, but in practice the hand and the wrist, are the most used, because they possess a great number of bones and epiphyses in development what allows the pursuit of the changes that happen through the years of the growth (Freitas et al. 2004; Jordan, 1979). They are also the most convenient areas to value the bone maturation, to be far from the gonads and to need less radiation (Jordán et al. 1987; Recalde Cortes et al. 1997).

The methods that are used to evaluate the growth potential of the left hand are: the TW2 that determines the bone age according to the maturation stages of each one of the bones; and the Grave and Brown that divides the process of maturation of the bones in nine stages of skeletal maturation. These two methods have disadvantage for the Orthodontics patients because the use of an additional X-ray, which is not carried out in the dental X rays machine, being necessary the patient's remission.

The current tendency in Orthodontics in the evaluation of the bone maturation is to reduce the number of X-rays to the strictly necessary ones (Bujaldón Daza et al., 1998), for that investigators exist as: Hassel and Farman (Hassel & Farman, 1995) that they try to develop some indexes of skeletal maturation with the profiles of the bodies of the cervical vertebras that appear in the lateral teleradiography of skull used for the orthodontist diagnostic. The advantages of using the cervical vertebras, it is centered in the reduction of radiographies to those that are subjected to the patients and for the easiness of consenting to the same ones (Ortiz et al., 2007)

Also in patient of Orthodontics with the objective of doing without of the X-ray of the hand that constitutes an additional exhibition to radiations, and it implies the use of a machine of rays X that is not used in a conventional way in Dentistry; the evaluation of the bone maturation has been used and of the growth potential through the development of the phalanges, that also has the purpose of simplifying the estimate, since alone the changes are analyzed at level of some phalanges, according to the relationship between the epiphysis and the diaphysis (Madhu et al., 2003).

Inside the diagnosis in Orthodontics, it is very important the evaluation of the growth potential, since most of the patients that require orthodontist treatment, are in a period of active growth, and with the treatment it can modify the facial growth, well be braking it, accelerating it or forward a normal vector (Tedaldi et al, 2007). According to Proffit (Proffit, 1994) it is not possible to modify a growth that is not taking place, and if a functional apparatus is placed on a patient that is not growing, the obtained result will be almost totally a dental mobilization.

The children with maxillary discrepancies usually benefit from the application of techniques to modify the growth. Since the bones of the face, and in particular the maxillary ones, suffer spontaneous changes during the different phases of growth, before establishing a treatment to correct skeletal malocclusions, it is necessary to know the opportune moment to begin the same one, according to the growth potential that the patient presents, to make more efficient our therapy (Tedaldi et al., 2007, Proffit, 1994).

The guiding principle is that growth can only be modified when it is occurring (Proffit, 1994), there is the importance of knowing the growth potential that the patient presents, when we carry out the diagnosis of the skeletal problems. Keeping in mind these aspects motivates ourselves to determine in the same sample three appraisal methods of the growth potential (Method TW2, Serious method and Brown, and determination of the stages of maturation of the half phalange of the third finger), with the objective of to propose a simplified method to determine the growth potential in patient of Orthodontics.

3. Methodological design

A cross-sectional technological innovation research was conducted in the period of January 2004 to April 2007, in the Clinic of Orthodontics of Havana School of Dentistry, in a sample of 150 patients between 8 and 16 years of age. A sampling was used by quotas according to sex and age, being divided in two groups, 75 for each sex. The patients were selected with previous condition to present good state of general health; to have measures of weight and height, that were between 10 and 90 percentile, of the Cuban Score of Weight for Height (Gutiérrez Muñiz et al., 2006); absence of chronic illnesses; absence of oligodontias; absences of congenital malformations; that they didn't have treatment corrective of the spinal column ; the need for the characteristics of their malocclusion, the realization of a lateral teleradiography of skull to complete their diagnosis; and to have signed the informed consent in writing.

3.1 Variables

Were studied the variables: chronological age, bone age (TW2), sex, stages of skeletal maturation and stages of maturation of the middle phalanx of the third finger.

Chronological age: Was considered the decimal age (Jordán, 1979): For the calculation, we subtracted the boy's date of birth and the date of the exam. The numeral was provided by the last two digits of the year and the decimal fraction was looked for in the table of decimal age.

Bone age (TW2): Was calculated in dependence of the sum of the punctuation of each stage for Radius, Ulna and Fingers, according to the patterns of the Cuban population's bone maturation, for the method TW2 (Jiménez et al., 1987).

Sex: Female and male.

Stages of skeletal maturation: Was classified according to Grave and Brown's method in stages of the 1 at 9.

Stages of maturation of the middle phalanx of the third finger: Was classified according to the relationship among the epiphysis and the diaphysis in one of the following stages (Toledo, 2004):

a.   The epiphysis has smaller width than the diaphysis.
b.   The epiphysis has the same width with the diaphysis.
c.   The epiphysis surrounds the diaphysis by way of cap.
d.   Begins the coalition between the epiphysis and the diaphysis.
e.   Where the epiphysis becomes ossified with the diaphysis.

3.2 Ethical aspects

With all the patients that participated in the investigation and their parents, an interview was conducted before the beginning of that, where they were explained on what it consisted with the study, frequency, evaluation type and the radiological protection measures that would be taken for not damaging the patient's health. If they agreed, the patients and their parents should sign the informed consent, approving their holding in the study.

3.3 Technical and procedures of obtaining the information

3.3.1 For the determination of: The bone age and the stages of skeletal maturation

Firstly you proceeded to each observer's training in the appraisal methods of the studied maturation. The information was picked up and analyzed by two residents and two specialists of Orthodontics, each resident and each specialist determined in the same sample, one of the two methods of study of the maturation analyzed in this investigation (method TW2 and method of Grave and Brown).

To each patient was made the clinical history of Orthodontics and was realized an radiographic of the left hand (Fig. 1) where they were determined: the bone age for the method TW2 (Jiménez et al, 1987) and the stages of skeletal maturation for the method of Grave and Brown (Tedaldi et al. 2007).

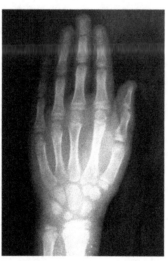

Fig. 1. Radiographic of the left hand.

The radiographic of the left hand was realized with the same regulations that the utilized ones in the National Study of Growth and Human Development in Cuba, carried out by Jordan (Jordán, 1979).

Each radiographic of the left hand was evaluated by the resident and the specialist in a first observation and in three weeks later in a second observation; that is to say a total of four times to calculate the variability inter and intra observant. The cases where discrepancy existed they were studied again to obtain the final results.

3.3.2 To determine the stages of skeletal maturation of the middle phalanx of the third finger of the left hand

In a paper of size Letter (21,59 cm. x 27,94 cm.), at a distance of 10 cm. of the superior margin and 10 cm. of the left margin, the contour of a film dental standard, Kodak marks, of 41x31 mm. was traced, and it was clipped by the traced area, being an opening in the paper with the dimensions of the dental film.

The paper was placed on the X-rays of the left hand of the 150 studied patients, it was made coincide the opening of the paper on the union between the middle phalanx and the proximal phalanx of the third finger and it was placed on a fixed negatoscope (Fig. 2).

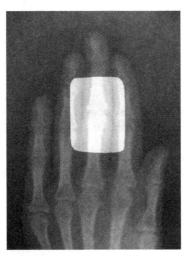

Fig. 2. Placement of the prepared paper on the union between the middle phalanx and the proximal phalanx of the third finger, in the radiographic of the left hand.

The analysis of the radiographic was carried out using a compass to measure the bone size in the middle phalanx and the maturation stage was classified with A to E, according to the classification proposed by Toledo (Toledo, 2004). With this procedure it was possible to locate each patient evaluated in a stage of maturation of the middle phalanx of the third finger, the same one was carried out by the main investigator and a specialist in Orthodontics, member of the investigation team, in two different opportunities to calculate the variability intra and inter observant.

3.4 Technical and procedures of elaboration and analysis

The information was stored in a data base automated in the system Excel, of the package Office 2003 on Windows XP professional and for the prosecution of the results the statistical packages SPSS version 11.5 and STATISTICA version 6.1 were used.

To calculate the variability intra and inter observant in the studied methods, the coefficient Kappa was applied (Begole, 2003).

The percentage was used for the qualitative variables and for the quantitative variables the arithmetic mean like measure summary and the standard deviation like variation measure (Bayarre et al. 2005).

You prove statistics employees: The association grade was calculated among the quantitative variables by means of the lineal correlation coefficient of Pearson (Begole, 2003) and the association grade among the variables in ordinal scales by means of the correlation coefficient of ranges of Spearman (Begole, 2003). To calculate the concordance among the results obtained in the studied methods, the coefficient Kappa was applied (Begole, 2003).

In all the used statistical tests, the used level of significance was of 0.05.

The results were presented in tables designed to the effect.

4. Results

In this epigraph the main results are presented, it contains the analysis of 6 tables.

The analysis of the variability intra and inter observant, their agreement was evaluated regarding the methods studied by means of an index Kappa. With relationship to the variability intra observant, that is to say, the level of discrepancy with regard to the valuations of oneself after three weeks, discrepancies didn't exist, in the three valued methods, being the agreement of 1,000 in the 150 cases, in each one of the methods. With relationship to the variability inter observant, that is to say, the level of discrepancy with regard to the valuations among the two observants, discrepancies didn't exist among these, being the agreement of 1,000 in the 150 cases, for these three methods.

4.1 Determination according to sex and chronological age of: The bone age, the stages of skeletal maturation and the stages of maturation of the middle phalanx of the third finger

4.2 Identification of the relationship among the bone age and: The chronological age, the stages of skeletal maturation and the stages of maturation of the middle phalanx of the third finger

Table 1 shows the arithmetic mean and the standard deviation of the chronological age and the bone age, calculated by the method TW2, according to groups of ages in the feminine sex, were found that in the groups of ages that were between the 8,00 and the 12,99 years and of 15.00 to 16.99 years, the bone age was bigger than the chronological one, being smaller in the remaining groups of ages. The coefficient of lineal correlation of Pearson among the bone age (TW2) and the chronological one presented a value of 0,977; that which signifies a very strong positive correlation, highly significant (p <0,010).

Group of Ages	Chronological age		Bone age (TW2)	
	X_1	DE_1	X_2	DE_2
8,00-8,99	8,38	0,33	8,72	1,22
9,00-9,99	9,87	0,17	10,55	0,47
10,00-10,99	10,53	0,33	10,58	0,98
11,00-11,99	11,58	0,24	12,36	0,47
12,00-12,99	12,75	0,20	13,32	0,89
13,00-13,99	13,42	0,28	12,57	0,73
14,00-14,99	14,86	0,01	14,78	0,46
15,00-16,99	15,19	0,14	15,20	0,70

r= 0,977 p = 0,000 n =75
r (lineal correlation coefficient of Pearson among bone age (TW2) and chronological age).

Table 1. Arithmetic mean (X) and standard deviation (DE) of chronological age and bone age (TW2) by groups of age in females.

Table 2 shows the arithmetic mean and the standard deviation of the chronological age and the bone age calculated by the method TW2 according to groups of ages in the masculine sex, it was found that in the groups of ages that were between 8,00 and 12,99 years, the bone age was smaller than the chronological one, being bigger starting from 13,00 years. The coefficient of lineal correlation of Pearson among the bone age (TW2) and the chronological one presented a value of 0,983; that which signifies a very strong positive correlation, highly significant (p <0,010).

Group of Ages	Chronological age		Bone age (TW2)	
	X_1	DE_1	X_2	DE_2
8,00-9,99	8,98	0,66	8,94	0,97
10,00-10,99	10,83	0,03	9,96	0,87
11,00-11,99	11,40	0,35	11,35	0,92
12,00-12,99	12,66	0,35	12,36	0,94
13,00-13,99	13,44	0,20	14,24	0,47
14,00-14,99	14,52	0,20	14,83	0,37
15,00-15,99	15,55	0,20	15,61	0,48
16,00-16,99	16,40	0,20	16,46	0,61

r = 0,983 p = 0,000 n =75
r (lineal correlation coefficient of Pearson among bone age (TW2) and chronological age).

Table 2. Arithmetic mean (X) and standard deviation (DE) of chronological age and bone age (TW2) by groups of age in males.

Table 3 shows the arithmetic mean and the standard deviation of the chronological age and the bone age (TW2) according to stages of skeletal maturation and sex, it was found that in each maturation stage, the averages of the chronological age were smaller in the feminine sex than in the masculine one. With relationship to the bone age calculated by the method TW2, in the feminine sex the averages of the same one went superior to those of the chronological age, in all the studied stages, however, in the masculine sex the bone age overcame the chronological one in the stages 4, 5, 6 and 8. The stages 4 and 5 are those of more clinical significance, belonged together with the chronological ages of 11,35 and 11,77 years in the feminine sex and 13,76 and 13,82 years in the masculine one and with the bone ages of 11,78 and 12,34 years in the feminine sex and of 14,20 and 14,57 years in the masculine one. It was observed that the females were earlier in their maturation stages than the males and that the stages advanced as it increased the chronological age and the bone age of the patients, in both sexes. The coefficient of correlation of ranges of Spearman among the bone age (TW2) and the stages of skeletal maturation presented a value of 0,855 in the feminine sex and 0,903 in the masculine one, both sexes showed a positive correlation, very significant (p <0,010). In the studied sample they were not patient in the stage 9.

Stages of skeletal maturation	Chronological age				Bone age (TW2)			
	Female		Male		Female		Male	
	X_1	DE_1	X_1	DE_1	X_2	DE_2	X_2	DE_2
1	8,59	0,66	11,38	1,34	8,97	1,25	10,66	1,11
2	10,06	0,54	11,61	0,87	10,25	0,71	10,50	1,20
3	11,63	1,35	11,71	0,65	11,82	0,84	10,50	0,89
4	11,35	1,71	13,76	0,80	11,78	1,18	14,20	0,14
5	11,77	1,18	13,82	1,13	12,34	0,99	14,57	0,72
6	13,34	0,97	14,96	0,97	13,77	0,79	15,46	0,54
7	15,31	0,17	16,35	0,48	15,45	0,07	16,08	0,62
8	14,24	0,98	16,25	0,23	14,45	1,03	16,56	0,28

Sex Female rho= 0,855 p = 0,000 n =75
Sex Male rho= 0,903 p = 0,000 n =75
rho (Correlation coefficient of Spearman among bone age (TW2) and stages of skeletal maturation.

Table 3. Arithmetic mean (X) and standard deviation (DE) of chronological age and bone age (TW2) by stages of skeletal maturation and sex.

Table 4 shows arithmetic mean and the standard deviation of the chronological age and the bone age (TW2) according to stages of maturation of the middle phalanx of the third finger and sex, it was found that in all the maturation stages the averages of the chronological age were smaller in the feminine sex than in the masculine one. In feminine sex the bone age overcame the chronological one in all the stages and in the masculine one in the stages B, C and E. The stage C (cap stage), it happened that 11,77 year-old chronological age and the bone one of 12,34 years, with a standard deviation of 1,18 and 0,99 years respectively in the females, while in the males, went to the 13,82 years and 14,57 years, with a standard deviation of 1,13 and 0,72 years respectively. It was observed that the females were earlier in their maturation stages than the males. The coefficient of correlation of ranges of Spearman among the bone age (TW2) and the stages of maturation of the middle phalanx of the third finger presented a value of 0,888 in the feminine sex and 0,921 in the masculine one, both sexes showed a positive correlation, very significant (p <0,010).

Stages of maturation of the middle phalanx of the third finger	Chronological age				Bone age (TW2)			
	Female		Male		Female		Male	
	X_1	DE_1	X_1	DE_1	X_2	DE_2	X_2	DE_2
A	8,59	0,66	11,38	1,34	8,97	1,25	10,66	1,11
B	11.55	1.4	13.06	0.71	11.52	0.92	13.25	0.92
C	11,77	1,18	13,82	1,13	12,34	0,99	14,57	0,72
D	13.83	1.23	15.93	0.86	13.59	1.17	15.7	0.63
E	14.24	0.98	16.25	0.23	14.45	1.03	16.56	0.28

Sex Female rho= 0,888 p = 0,000 n =75
Sex Male rho= 0,921 p = 0,000 n =75
rho (Correlation coefficient of Spearman among bone age (TW2) and stages of maturation of the middle phalanx of the third finger

Table 4. Arithmetic mean (X) and standard deviation (DE) of chronological age and bone age (TW2) by stages of maturation of the middle phalanx of the third finger and sex.

4.3 Identification of concordance between the studied methods

Table 5 shows the percentages of females according to the stages of skeletal maturation and stages of maturation of the middle phalanx of the third finger, it was found that in the stage of skeletal maturation 1, 100,00% was in the stage A of maturation of the middle phalanx of the third finger; in the stages 2, 3 and 4, 100% was in the stage B of the phalanx; in the stage 5, 100% was in the C; in the 6 and the 7, 100,00% was in the stage D and in the stage 8, 100,00% was in the stage E of the phalanx. The coefficient of concordance Kappa between the stages of skeletal maturation and the stages of maturation of the middle phalanx of the third finger, presented a value of 1,000 that which evidenced a perfect concordance, very significant (p <0.010).

Stages of skeletal maturation	Total	Stages of maturation of the middle phalanx of the third finger									
		A		B		C		D		E	
		#	%	#	%	#	%	#	%	#	%
1	12	12	100,00	-	-	-	-	-	-	-	-
2	8	-	-	8	100,00	-	-	-	-	-	-
3	10	-	-	10	100,00	-	-	-	-	-	-
4	4	-	-	4	100,00	-	-	-	-	-	-
5	15	-	-	-	-	15	100,00	-	-	-	-
6	6	-	-	-	-	-	-	6	100,00	-	-
7	2	-	-	-	-	-	-	2	100,00	-	-
8	18	-	-	-	-	-	-	-	-	18	100,00

Coefficient Kappa = 1,000 p=0,000 n=75

Table 5. Percentage of females according to stages of skeletal maturation and stages of maturation of the middle phalanx of the third finger.

Table 6 shows the percentages of males according to the stages of skeletal maturation and stages of maturation of the middle phalanx of the third finger, it was found that in the stage of skeletal maturation 1, 100,00% was in the stage A of maturation of the middle phalanx of the third finger; in the stages 2, 3 and 4, 100% was in the stage B of the phalanx; in the stage 5, 100% was in the C; in the 6 the biggest percent was in the D (75,00); in the 7, 100,00% was in the stage D and in the stage 8, 100,00% was in the stage E of the phalanx. The coefficient of concordance Kappa between the stages of skeletal maturation and the stages of maturation of the middle phalanx of the third finger, presented a value of 0,964; that which evidenced a high concordance, very significant (p <0.010).

Stages of skeletal maturation	Total	Stages of maturation of the middle phalanx of the third finger									
		A		B		C		D		E	
		#	%	#	%	#	%	#	%	#	%
1	15	15	100,00	-	-	-	-	-	-	-	-
2	11	-	-	11	100,00	-	-	-	-	-	-
3	12	-	-	12	100,00	-	-	-	-	-	-
4	2	-	-	2	100,00	-	-	-	-	-	-
5	20	-	-	-	-	20	100,00	-	-	-	-
6	8	-	-	-	-	2	25,00	6	75,00	-	-
7	5	-	-	-	-	-	-	5	100,00	-	-
8	2	-	-	-	-	-	-	-	-	2	100,00

Coefficient Kappa = 0,964 p=0,000 n=75

Table 6. Percentage of males according to stages of skeletal maturation and stages of maturation of the middle phalanx of the third finger.

5. Discussion

In this epigraph, one discussed the most important results and they were compared with the results of other investigations, with foundations starting from the revised bibliography.

With relationship to the variability intra and inter observant results were completely coincident in the three studied methods. The author considers that the results are due to the previous training of the investigators in each one of the studied evaluation methods.

With relationship to the variability intra observant and inter observant in the analysis of the stage of maturation of the middle phalanx of the third finger, coincidence existed among the four carried out observations. The author considers that the results are due to the simplification of this method, since in the same alone the changes are analyzed at level of a single phalanx.

In the studied sample, the bone age of the patients, calculated through the method TW2, didn't coincide with the chronological age. These results coincide with those of Malavé and Rojas (Malavé & Rojas, 2000) whom they outlined that, the chronological age is not a good indicator of the level of an individual's bone maturation.

In the three methods of study of the analyzed maturation, it was found that the females matured before the males of their same age. These results coincide with studies carried out for Grave and Townsend (Grave & Townsend, 2003), Demirjian et al. (Demirjian et al, 1985) and Liversidge and Speechly (Liversidge & Speechly, 2001), who they find that, the females mature more early than the males, that which is important to consider in the general evaluation of the orthodontist patient.

There were a positive, very significant correlation (p <0,010) among the bone age (TW2) and the stages of skeletal maturation in both sexes (rho = 0,855 for the females and rho = 0,903 for the males). These results coincide with other carried out studies (Moore et al., 1990; Uysal et al., 2006).

In the analysis of the stages of maturation of the half phalange of the third finger it was found that the females were earlier in their maturation stages than the males. These results belong together with those obtained in other methods analyzed in this investigation and they coincide with those of Hägg and Taranger (Hägg & Taranger, 1980a, 1980b, 1982) who they find that, the females mature early, that which is important to consider in the planning of the orthodontist treatment.

The coefficient of correlation of Spearman among the bone age (TW2) and the stages of maturation of the middle phalanx of the third finger showed positive, very significant correlations (p <0,010); in both sexes (0,888 in the feminine one and 0, 921 in the masculine one). These results coincide with other studies that analyze the bone maturation through the development of the phalanges: Leite et al. (Leite et al., 1987) they carry out a longitudinal study, through which value the age skeletal analyzing the first one, second and third fingers of the hand, in a sample of 19 males radiographies and 20 females whose radiographic of the annual hand-wrist had taken from the 10 to the 16 years for the girls and of 12 to 18 years for the males and they find that although differences exist between the analysis of the total hand and that of the three fingers, the method of the three fingers never strays of that of the hand-wrist for more than 2.89 months for the males with a minimum deviation of 0.32 months and for the females, the maximum deviation was of 4.45 months with a minimum of 1.55 months. They also find that the maximum deviations happen during the time of coalition of the epiphysis with the diaphysis when the growth is coming closer to their finalization and consequently they are not of clinical importance. These authors conclude that the advantage of the use of the method of the three fingers is that they can incorporate in the lateral teleradiography, eliminating this way the necessity of other radiographies.

Shigemi Goto et al. (Shigemi Goto & Yamada Miyazawa, 1996) carry out a study in which analyze the ossification of the distal phalanx of the first finger like an indicator of maturity for the initiation of the orthodontist treatment in 2 Japanese women with Class III malocclusion, where they conclude that the determination of the phases of maturation skeletal of the distal phalanx of the first finger, it can be a quick and useful clinical method, to evaluate the potential of residual growth in the cases of Class III.

Rossi et al. (Rossi et al., 1999) carry out a study in 72 feminine patients with ages understood between 8 and 13 years of age, where they analyze the proximal phalanx of the first finger and they find that in the patients that were in the epiphysis stage C, they were next to the peak of maximum speed of growth pubertal.

In relation of the concordance between the stages of skeletal maturation and the stages of maturation of the middle phalanx of the third finger, in the studied sample a high concordance existed, very significant (p <0,010) in both sexes, being perfect in the feminine sex (1,000). That which coincides with other carried out studies: Rajagopal and Sudhanshu (Rajagopal & Sudhanshu, 2002) carry out a study with the objective of determining the dependability of using radiographic of the middle phalanx of the third finger as an indicator of skeletal maturation, in a sample of 75 girls and 75 children, between the 9 and 17 years of age; where they compare the stages of maturation of the cervical vertebras, and the stages of maturation of the middle phalanx of the third finger and they conclude that the assessment of the growth puberal based on the observations of the middle phalanx of the third finger observed by means of standard X-rays, is an useful method and it has as advantages: the smallest exhibition to the X rays and that X rays supplementary machine is not needed.

Madhu et al. (Madhu et al., 2003) carry out a study with the objective of obtaining a unique and simple method to determine the skeletal maturation using the stages of development of the middle phalanx of the third finger that one observes in a radiographic, taken with a conventional X ray dental machine; in a sample of 67 patients, 35 males between 10 and 18 years of age and 32 females between 8 and 16 years. To the patients they carry out them lateral teleradiographies of skull and an X-ray of the area of the middle phalanx of the third finger, where they determine the stages of maturation of the cervical vertebras of the patients in previous stages to the peak puberal, patient that were in the peak of growth puberal and patient in those that it had already happened the peak of growth puberal and the stages of the middle phalanx of the third finger are classified in 3 stages: patient in the previous period to reach the peak pubertal of growth, patient that are in the period of growth pubertal and those patients that the period of growth pubertal had passed. These authors find agreement among the results obtained in the analysis of the cervical vertebras and of the middle phalanx of the third finger and they conclude that the analysis of the maturation of the middle phalanx of the third finger, is an alternative method that can be used to determine the skeletal maturation of the children in growth.

Ozer et al. (Ozer et al., 2006) carry out a study in 150 masculine patients, with ages understood among 9 and 19 years that were in orthodontist treatment, with the purpose of determining the correlation between the index of maturation of the cervical vertebras and the stages of maturation of the middle phalanx of the third finger, for that which they carry out lateral teleradiography of skull and X-rays of the middle phalanx of the third finger of the left hand, finding high correlation coefficients between the stages of vertebral maturation and those of the phalanges. They conclude that the middle phalanx of the third finger can be used in the evaluation of the skeletal maturation of the patients.

From the clinical point of view in the planning of an orthodontist treatment, we should consider if the patient has begun the spurt of pubertal growth, if this is happening in that moment or if it has concluded (Tedaldi, 2007). With the analysis of the stages of maturation of the middle phalanx of the third finger, visualized in an X-ray of 41 x 31 mm., is possible to determine: if the patient has not reached the spurt of pubertal growth (Stage A), if it is next or this event already began (B), if it is in its maximum peak (C) or if it is in the descending curve of growth pubertal (D and E) (Toledo Mayarí & Otaño Lugo, 2010).

Due to the high correlation coefficient found in this sample, between the stages of maturation of the middle phalanx of the third finger and the bone age in both sexes, as well as to the high concordance found in this study, among the evaluation of the maturation through the left hand and the analysis of the middle phalanx of the third finger, which was perfect in the feminine sex, and considering the current tendency in Orthodontics of reducing the number of radiations, we propose inside the diagnosis for the evaluation of the potential growth of the patients, the realization of an X-ray of 41 x 31 mm. of the middle phalanx of the third finger of the left hand (Fig. 3), with the following requirements:

An auxiliary table will be used, where the radiography of 41x31 mm. will be placed, with the vertical bigger axis coinciding with the same position of the phalanx and with the active face in front of the focus. The radiograph will be located on the union between the middle and proximal phalanx of the third finger of the left hand, with the coincident located reference point with the proximal phalanx. The focus will be centered in perpendicular sense to the table, with an angle of 90 °, at a distance focus film, using short cone, of 11 cm. with a time of exhibition of 0,5 second. The calibration of the machine will be of 110 volt / 10 MA / seg. They will take all the measures of protection radiological established (Ugarte et al., 2004) and a dental machine of X rays and dental films standard of 41x31mm., Kodak marks. The one revealed will be executed looking for soft revealed low contrasts.

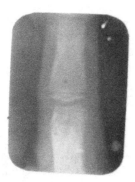

Fig. 3. Radiographic of middle phalanx of the third finger.

The author considers that, in the patients, it is not necessary to carry out a lateral teleradiography of skull, the evaluation of the potential of growth, inside the diagnosis in Orthodontics, one can make through the stages of maturation of the middle phalanx of the third finger of the left hand, which contributes the following benefits:

It constitutes a simplified method that can be applied in any service of Orthodontics and it allows planning for the treatment of orthodontics in dependence of the potential of growth which the patient presents that makes more efficient therapy.

It allows bigger efficiency and decrease of the costs and it can be carried out in the dental X rays machine, for what includes relative savings to the depreciation of the machine of X-rays and the energy consumption.

They diminish the quantity from radiations to those that are exposed to the patients and the auxiliary personnel (technicians in radiology), as well as, the radiations in the local where the radiographies were taken.

6. Conclusions

The evaluation of the potential of growth that the patients of Orthodontics present can be made by means of the realization of radiography of the middle phalanx of the third finger of the left hand.

In the three certain methods, it was found that the females mature before the males of their same age.

It existed a high correlation and concordance among the studied methods of determination of the potential growth.

The substitution of the radiography of the left hand, for the radiography of the middle phalanx of the third finger, allows the realization of that in the own service of Dentistry, with the benefits that it reports as for the patient's better attention.

The results of this study prove the hypothesis formulated and constituted part of the Thesis in option to PhD degree in Dentistry of the author.

7. Acknowledgment

This research project would not have been possible without the support of many people. The author wishes to express her gratitude to her mother Dr. Zoila Gúdula Mayarí Cano, who introduced her into Dentistry, her tutor, Prof. PhD. Rigoberto Otaño Lugo of blessed memory who was abundantly helpful and offered invaluable assistance, support and guidance. Deepest gratitude also goes to all the members of the investigation team, without whose knowledge and assistance this study would not have been successful.

8. References

Abreu Suárez, G., González Valdés, J A., Jordán Rodríguez, J. & Chiong Molina, D. (1995). Growth and bone maturation in asthmatic children. *Rev Cub Aliment Nutr*, Vol.9, No.2, pp. 106-12.

Bayarre, H. et al. (2005). *Descriptive Statistic and statistic of Health*, Editorial Medical Sciences, Havana City, Cuba

Begole, EA. (2003). Statistic for the orthodontist, In: *Orthodontics. General and Technical principles*, Graber TM, Vanarsdall (h) RL, 3a ed., Pan-American Medical editorial, Buenos Aires, Argentina.

Björk, A. & Helm, S. (1967). Prediction of age of maximum puberal growth in body height. *Angle Orthod*, Vol.37, No.2, pp. 134 – 43.

Bujaldón Daza, JM., Rodríguez Argáiz. R. & Bujaldón Daza, AL. (1998). Study preliminary about the validity of the index of maturation of the cervical vertebras as diagnostic tool in the orthodontist planning, *RCOE*, Vol.3, No.8, pp 751-760.

Cannut Brusola, JA. (1988). *Clinical orthodontics*, Scientific and Technical editions, S.A., Barcelona, España.

Cattani, A. (2003). *Studies Health and the adolescent's development. Module I: Lesson 1. Growth and development puberal during the adolescence*, [on-line article], 11.05.2005.Available from: http://escuela.med.puc.cl/paginas/OPS/Curso/Lecciones/Leccion01/M1L1Leccio n.html.

Ceglia, A. (2005). Indicative of maturation of the bone, dental and morphological age. *Revista Latinoamericana de Ortodoncia y Odontopediatría*. [online], 03.02.2007; Available from: http://www.ortodoncia.ws/publicaciones/2005/indicadores_maduracion_edad_o sea_dental_morfologica.asp .

Cha, KS. (2003). Skeletal changes of maxillary protraction in patients exhibiting skeletal class III malocclusion: a comparison of three skeletal maturation groups. *Angle Orthod*, Vol.73, No.1, pp. 2635.

Demirjian, A., Bushchang, PH., Tanguay, R. & Patterson, DK. (1985). Interrelationships of measure of somatic, skeletal dental and sexual maturity. *Am J Orthod Dentofac Orthop*, Vol.88, pp. 433- 8.

Edilmar, M., Tavano, O., & Carvalho, IM. (2005). Cervical vertebral like estimate do grow and development in patient with lip-palatal fissures. *Salusvita* Vol.24, No.1, pp. 11-28.

Fiani, E. (1998). Indicative of maturation skeletal, bone, dental and morphological age. *Rev Cub Ortod*, Vol.13, No.2, pp. 121 – 125.

Fishman, LS. (1982). Radiographic evaluation of skeletal maturation. A clinically oriented method based on hand-wrist films. *Angle Orthod*, Vol.52, pp. 88-111.

Freitas, D., Maia, J., Beunen, G., Lefevre, J., Claessens, A., Marques, A. et al. (2004). Skeletal maturity and socio-economic status in Portuguese children and youths: the Madeira growth study. *Ann Hum Biol*, Vol.31, No.4, pp. 408-20.

Gandini, P., Mancini, M. & Andreani, F.(2006). A comparison of hand-wrist bone and cervical vertebral analyses in measuring skeletal maturation. *Angle Orthod*, Vol.76, No.6, pp. 984-9.

Geran, RG., McNamara, JJr., Baccetti, T., Franchi, L. & Shapiro, L. (2006). A prospective long-term study on the effects of rapid maxillary expansion in the early mixed dentition. *Am J Orthod Dentofac Orthop*, Vol.129, No.5, pp. 454-62.

Grave, K. & Townsend, G. (2003). Cervical vertebral maturation as a predictor of the adolescent growth spurt. *Aust Orthod J*, Vol.19, No.2, pp. 44-47.

Greulich, WW. & Pyle, SI. (1959). *Radiographic Atlas of Skeletal Development of the Hand and Wrist*. 2nd ed., Oxford University Press, London, England.

Gupta, S. (1995). Assessment of puberty growth spurt in boys and girls: a dental radiographic method. *J Indian Soc Pedod Prev Dent*, Vol.13, No.1, pp.4 – 9.

Gutiérrez Muñiz, JA., Berdasco Gómez, A., Esquivel Lauzurique, M., Jiménez Hernández, JM., Posada Lima, E., Romero del Sol, JM. et al. (2006). Growth and Development. In: *Pediatrics*, Collective of Authors, T1. [online]. 14.02.2007. Editorial Medical Sciences; Havana, Cuba. Available from:
http://www.bvs.sld.cu/libros_texto/pediatria_tomoi/parteii_cap06.pdf.

Hägg, U. & Taranger, J. (1982). Maturation indicators and the pubertal growth spurt. *Am J Orthod Dentofac Orthop*, Vol.82, No.4, pp. 299 – 309.

Hägg, U. & Taranger, J. (1980). Menarche and voice change as indicators of the pubertal growth spurt. *Acta Odontol Scand*, Vol.38, pp. 170 – 86.

Hägg, U. & Taranger, J. (1980). Skeletal stages of the hand and wrist as indicators of the pubertal growth spurt. *Acta Odontol Scand*, Vol.38, pp. 187 – 200.

Hassel, B. & Farman, AG. (1995). Skeletal maturation evaluation using cervical vertebrae. *Am J Orthod Dentofac Orthop*, Vol.107, pp. 58-66.

Izaguirre de Espinoza, I., Macías de Tomei, C., Castañeda de Gómez, M. &, Méndez Castellano H. (2003). Atlas Venezuelan bone maturation. *An Venez Nutr*, Vol.16, No.1, pp. 23-30.

Jiménez Hernández, JM., Romero del Sol, JM., Rubén Quesada, M., Barrera Yanes, R, Berdasco Gómez, A. &, Jordán Rodríguez, J. (1986). Study of bone maturation by sex and race. *Rev Cub Ped*, Vol.58, No.5, pp. 533-45.

Jiménez, JM., Romero, JM., Barrera, R., Rúben, M., Berdasco, A. & Jordán, J. (1987). *Patron of Cuban population's bone maturation*. ISCMH, Havana City, Cuba.

Jordán, RJ. (1979). *Human Development*, Editorial Scientific-technique, Havana, Cuba.

Jordán J., Berdasco, A., & J iménez, JM. (1987). *Bone maturation. Method TW2*, ISCMH, Havana City, Cuba

Leite, HR., O'Reilly, MT. & Close, J. (1987). Skeletal age assessment with first, second and third fingers. *Am J Orthod Dentofac Orthop*; Vol.92, pp 492-8.

Liversidge, HM. & Speechly, T. (2001). Growth of permanent mandibular teeth of British children aged 4 to 9 years. *Ann Hum Biol*, Vol.28, No.3, pp. 256-62.

Madhu, S., Hedge, AM. & Munshi, AK. (2003). The developmental stages of the middle phalanx of the third finger (MP3): a sole indicator in assessing the skeletal maturity? *J Clin Pediatr Dent*, Vol.27, No.2, pp.149-56.

Malavé, Y. & Rojas, I. (2000). Análisis Carpal como Indicador de Maduración Ósea. *Acta Odontol Venez* [online] 2000, Vol.30, No.3, pp.4-9. Available from http://www2.scielo.org.ve/scielo.php?script=sci_arttext&pid=S0001-63652000000300002&lng=en&nrm=iso .

Mayoral, J. & Mayoral, G. (1990). *Orthodontics: Fundamental principles and practice*. 6a ed., Labor S.A., Barcelona, Spain.

Moore, RN., Moyer, BA. & DuBois, LM. (1990). Skeletal maturation and craniofacial growth. *Am J Orthod Dentofac Orthop*, Vol.98, pp.33-40.

Nanda, R. (1955). The rate of growth of several facial components measured from serial cefalometric roentgenograms. *Am J Orthod Dentofac Orthop*, Vol.41, pp.129-141.

Ortega, AI., Haiter-Neto, F., Bovi Ambrosano, GM., Bóscolo, FN., Almeida, SM. &, Spinelli Casanova, M. (2006). Comparison of TW2 and TW3 skeletal age differences in a Brazilian population. *J Appl Oral Sci*. [online]. 27.09.2007. Vol.14, No.2, Available from: http://www.scielo.br/scielo.php?script=sci_arttext&pid=S1678-77572006000200014 .

Ortiz, M., Godoy, S., Fuenmayor, D., Farias, M., Quirós, O., Rondón, S. & Harry, L. (2007). Method of bone maturation of the cervical vertebras, in patient of the Graduate of Orthodontics Interceptiva, UGMA-2006. *Revista Latinoamericana de Ortodoncia y Odontopediatría* [online]. 29.06.2007. Available from: http://www.ortodoncia.ws/publicaciones/2007/maduracion_osea_vertebras_cervicales.asp .

Ozer, T., Kama, JD. &, Ozer, SY. (2006). A practical method for determining pubertal growth spurt. *Am J Orthod Dentofac Orthop*, Vol.130, No. 2, pp. 131-6.

Padrós, E. & Creus, M. (2002). Revision of the methods to study the growth craniofacial in orthodontics. *Ortod Clínic*, Vol.5, No. 2, pp. 100-116.

Paesano, PL., Vigone, MC., Siragusa, V., Chiumello, G., DelMaschio, A. & Mora, S (1998). Assessment of skeletal maturation in infants: comparison between two methods in hypothyroid patients. *Pediatr Radiol*, Vol.28, pp. 622-26.

Pancherz H. & Hägg V. (1985). Dentofacial orthopedic in relation to somatic maturation: An analysis of 7 consecutive cases treated with the Herbst appliance. *Am J Orthod Dentofac Orthop*, Vol.88, pp. 273 – 87.

Peluffo, PL. (2001). Indicators of maturation. Bone age and cervical vertebrae. *Rev Odont Interdis*, Vol.11, No. 3, pp. 9-15.

Proffit, WR. (1994). *Orthodontics: Theory and practice*. 2a ed., Mosby- Doyma Libros, S. A., Madrid, Spain.

Quirós Álvarez, OJ. (2006). *Base Bio mechans and Clinical Applications on Interceptive Orthodontics*. Actualidades Médico Odontológicas Latinoamericanas, Caracas, Venezuela.

Quirós Álvarez, OJ. (2000). *Manual of Maxillary Functional Orthopedics and Interceptive Orthodontics*. Actualidades Médico Odontológicas Latinoamericanas, Caracas, Venezuela.

Rajagopal, R. & Sudhanshu, K. A. (2002). Comparison of modified MP3 stages and the cervical vertebrae as growth indicators. *J Clin Orthod*, Vol.7, pp. 398-406.

Rakosi, T. & Jonas, I. (1992). *Atlas of Maxillary Orthopedics. Diagnostic*. Scientific and Technical editions, S. A., Barcelona, Spain.

Recalde Cortes, C., López Santomauro, D. & Palleiro, AM. (1997). Hand radiography, their clinical value. CEDDU, Vol. VIII, No.1, pp. 51-67.

Rossi Rowdley, R., Sandro Gomes, A. & Pacheco Thomé, MC. (1999). Correlation among dental stages mineralization and estimative of skeletal maturation. *Ortodontia*, Vol. 32, No. 3, pp. 48-58.

San Roman, P., Palma, JC., Oteo, MD. & Nevado, E. (2002). Squeletal maturation determined by cervical vertebrae development. *Eur J Orthod*, Vol.24, pp. 303-11.

Shigemi Goto, A. & Yamada Miyazawa, N. (1996) Ossification of the distal phalanx of the first digit as a maturity indicator for initiation of orthodontic treatment of Class III malocclusion in Japanese women. *Am J Orthod Dentofac Orthop*, Vol.110, pp. 490-501.

Spinelli Casanova, M., Ortega, AI., Haiter-Neto, F. & de Almeida, SM. (2006). Comparative Analyze bone maturation by Grave-Brown's method among conventional images and digitized. *Dental J Press Orthodon Facial Orthop* [online]. 22.06.2007, Vol. 11, No. 5, pp. 104-109. Available from:
http://www.scielo.br/pdf/dpress/v11n5/a11v11n5.pdf .

Tanner, JM., Whitehouse, RH., Cameron, N., Marshall, WA., Healy, MJR., & Goldstein, H. (1983). *Assessment of skeletal maturity and prediction of adult height (TW2 method)*. 2nd ed.. Academic Press, London, England.

Tedaldi, J., Calderón, R., Mayora, L., Quirós, O., Farias, M., Rondón, S., et al. (2007). Maloclussions treatment according to the stage of maturation carpal. Bibliographical revision. *Revista Latinoamericana de Ortodoncia y Odontopediatría*. [online], 29.06.2007; Available from:
http://www.ortodoncia.ws/publicaciones/2007/tratamiento_maloclusiones.asp.

Toledo Mayarí, G. & Otaño Lugo, R. (2010). A simplified method to determine the potential growth in Orthodontics patients. *Rev Cubana Estomatol*, Vol.47, No.2, pp. 134-142.[online]. 23.09.2011. Available from:
http://scielo.sld.cu/pdf/est/v47n2/est02210.pdf .

Toledo Mayarí, G. & Otaño Lugo, R. (2010). Concordance among skeletal maturation stages and dental calcification stages. *Rev Cubana Estomatol*, Vol.47, No.2, pp. 207-214. [online]. 23.09.2011. Available from:
http://scielo.sld.cu/pdf/est/v47n2/est09210.pdf

Toledo Mayarí, G. & Otaño Lugo, R. (2010). Assessment of bone maturation in cervical vertebrae in Orthodontics patients. *Rev Cubana Estomatol*, Vol.47, No.3, pp. 326-335. [online]. 23.09.2011. Available from:
http://scielo.sld.cu/pdf/est/v47n3/est06310.pdf

Toledo, V. (2004). *Orthognatic Surgeon Simplification of the treatment Surgical Orthodontic in Adults.*, Amorca Caracas, Venezuela.

Ugarte Suárez, JC., Banasco Domínguez, J. & Ugarte Moreno, D. (2004). *Manual of Imagenology.* 2a ed., Editorial Medical Sciences, Havana City, Cuba.

Uysal, T., Ramoglu, IF., Basciftci, FA. & Sari, ZA. (2006). Chronologic age and skeletal maturation of the cervical vertebrae and hand-wrist: is there a relationship? *J Orthod Dentofac Orthop*, Vol.130, No.5, pp. 622-8.

7

Genetic Factors Affecting Facial Growth

James K. Hartsfield Jr.[1], Lorri Ann Morford[1] and Liliana M. Otero[1,2]
[1]University of Kentucky
[2]Pontificia Universidad Javeriana
[1]USA
[2]Colombia

1. Introduction

Malocclusion is the manifestation of complex genetic and environmental interactions on the development of the oral-facial region. Historically, orthodontists have been interested in genetics as a means to better understand why a patient has a particular occlusion, and to determine the best course of treatment for the malocclusion. The application of genetic information in treatment, however, has been hampered by several factors including: 1) the presumption that heritability studies have some clinical relevance to the individual patient, which they do not (Harris, 2008); 2) the presumption that whatever genetic factors may have contributed to the occlusion will also affect how the patient responds to treatment, which they may not; and 3) a lack of understanding to the extent at which genetic factors may interact with environmental factors (such as those created during orthodontic and dentofacial orthopedic treatments) to influence single gene (Mendelian) traits versus "Complex" traits which are more frequently observed in the clinic. (Hartsfield, 2011)

While it is essential to consider genetic factors when diagnosing the underlying cause for virtually all oral-facial anomalies and developmental variations, the importance of how genetic factors will affect the outcome of treatment is often not appreciated. Understanding the etiology of a malocclusion is important, e.g., if the patient is a thumb sucker, then that habit must stop. But in terms of etiology, the factors that influenced a malocclusion to develop may not be the same ones that will influence how the patient responds to treatment of that malocclusion. In addition, the patient's developmental stage during treatment is typically a later stage then when the basis of the malocclusion first formed. Although an environmental modification may alter the development of the phenotype at a particular moment, gross structural morphology, already present, may not change readily unless the environmental modification is sufficient to alter preexisting structure.(Buschang & Hinton, 2005) As every orthodontist knows, the ability of the practitioner to affect a change is dependent both on the time of intervention (treatment) and the patient's stage of development.

Knowing whether the cause of the problem is genetic has been cited as a factor in eventual outcome; that is, if the problem is genetic, then orthodontists may be limited in what they can do (or change), because of an intrinsic "predestination." This is a misapplication of genetics to clinical practice since most malocclusions we treat appear to not be the result of a single dominant (Mendelian) gene.(Mossey, 1999b) There are inappropriate uses of heritability estimates in the literature as a proxy for evaluating whether a malocclusion or some anatomic morphology is "genetic." This however has no relevance to the question. Regardless of the heritability estimate, there is not a yes or no answer. Heritability estimates only apply to the group that was studied and the environmental factors that they were exposed to up to that time. They do not necessarily apply to an individual at the time of the study, and are not predictive for an individual or the group in the future.(Harris, 2008) How genetic factors will influence the response to environmental factors, including treatment, and the long-term stability of its outcome as determined by genetic linkage or association studies, should be the greatest concern for the clinician as they are the only way leading to a better understanding of the genetic background of the individual patient in terms of their malocclusion and response to treatment.(Hartsfield, 2008) It is of critical importance in clinical practice to understand how genetic factors and their interaction with environmental factors may affect facial growth. The aim of this chapter is to review what is known about the genetic factors that affect facial growth with an emphasis on human studies involving malocclusion.

2. Genome, genotype, phenotype, modes of inheritance and epigenetics

An individual's **genome** is defined as the genetic information inherited from both of their parents. The information encoded in a patient's genome can influence growth and development when the coded information is converted into the form of **protein** (and/or regulatory molecules such as microRNAs (miRNAs)). This information is encoded by ~3.2 billion nucleotide base pairs (bps), comprised of adenine (A), thymine (T) , cytosine (C) and guanine (G) residues, that are organized into sequences on 23 pairs of chromosomes. Each individual has 22 pairs of **autosomal chromosomes** (chromosomes that exhibit the same copy number in both males and females) and 1 pair of **sex chromosomes** (XX or XY). One chromosome of each pair is inherited from the individual's mother and the other pair from their father. Collectively this genetic information is often referred to as a person's DNA or genetic code. Amazingly, the genetic sequences of all humans appear to be ~99.9% identical, and hence it is a mere 0.1% of the sequence information which codes for our individual differences.

It is estimated that the human genome is comprised of 25,000 genes (accounting for only ~2% of the entire genome), with the average gene length being ~3,000 bps of information. A **gene** is a specific sequence of information that provides the instructions for making a unique protein or set of related proteins. The location or "address" for any gene within a genome is called its **locus** (plural loci: i.e., referring to the physical location of more than one gene). A determination of the actual DNA code (A, T, C or G) for a specific location within a person's genome describes their **genotype** for that location. Since there is natural variation in the sequence of DNA, a specific gene at a locus can still vary among individuals and homologous chromosomes in the same individual. These different forms of the "same" gene are called **alleles**. When the alleles on homologous chromosome pairs are the same, they are said to be **homozygous**. When the alleles on homologous chromosome pairs are different, they are said to be **heterozygous**. The **mode of inheritance** describes how the genetic information is passed down one generation to the next.

Within a single individual, the majority of cells in the body will contain a complete copy of the genome the individual inherited from their parents. Only a small number of specialized cell types (e.g. mature erythrocytes, mature T- and B-cells of the immune system, sperm, and egg cells) eliminate a portion of inherited DNA to facilitate the cell's ability to perform a specialized function. Aside from these specialized cell types, most cells within an individual's body become (or differentiate into) a particular kind of cell (e.g. a muscle, nerve, or skin cell, etc…) or become part of a larger tissue or organ based upon the pattern of genes that are turned "on" or "off" within each cell. The process of turning a gene "on" is referred to as "gene expression" and most forms of gene expression lead to the production a protein or set of related proteins. Hence, a well differentiated cell like an osteoblast, does not become an osteoblast due to the presence of unique DNA codes found only is osteoblast cells or due to the loss of non-osteoblast related genetic information. An osteoblast becomes an osteoblast due to the genes and related proteins (or regulatory molecules) being expressed within the cell combined with the influence of any environmental factors that can alter these expression pattern(s).

The visible or measurable characteristics of an individual is their **phenotype**. A phenotype is determined based on the combination of: (1) the inherited genetic information being expressed by cells within the individual (e.g., the individual's genotype); (2) the environment in which the proteins (or regulatory molecules) are being expressed; and (3) any genotype-environment interactions that could influence protein (or regulatory molecule) expression or function. In contrast, a **trait** is a particular aspect or characteristic of the overall phenotype. An **inherited trait** is one that has the ability to be transferred from one generation to the next generation. A **syndrome** is a combination of traits that occur together in non random pattern that is different from the usual pattern.(Hartsfield & Bixler, 2011)

When the information in a single gene locus is essentially responsible for the development of a trait or syndrome, this trait or syndrome is said to be *monogenic*. If the gene locus is located on one of 22 autosomal chromosome pairs (chromosomes other than the X or Y sex chromosomes), and only one copy of a specific gene allele on the autosomal pair is sufficient to lead to the production of the trait or syndrome, then the individual is typically heterozygous for that allele and the effect on the inheritance pattern of the trait or syndrome is **autosomal dominant**. If the production of the trait or syndrome does not occur when only one copy of a particular allele is present at the locus on a paired set of autosomes, but does occur when two copies of that particular allele are present at the locus of a paired set of autosomes, then the inheritance pattern of the trait or syndrome is **autosomal recessive**. In this situation the "recessive" alleles are said to be homozygous.(Mossey, 1999a) This may be the case by having a common ancestor (inbreeding) in which the alleles are presumed to be identical, or by the random combination of alleles that although may not be of identical DNA sequence, still are operationally recessive.

The following are characteristic for **autosomal dominant inheritance**: (1) the trait or syndrome occurs in successive generations; (2) when an individual has the gene allele that results in the trait or syndrome, each child of theirs has a 50% chance of inheriting that gene allele; (3) males and females are equally likely to have the trait or syndrome; and (4) parents who do not have the trait or syndrome have offspring who do not have the trait or syndrome (see figure 1). However, there are notable caveats to these characteristics. Just because an individual has the "dominant" gene allele that would usually lead to the development of some particular trait or syndrome, such as Class III malocclusion, Treacher

Collins syndrome or Crouzon syndrome (a common craniosynostosis condition), the appearance of the trait or syndrome may "skip a generation" in what is called **non-penetrance** in the individual, or incomplete penetrance in a group of individuals who have the genotype but don't manifest the trait or syndrome.(Cruz et al., 2008; Everett et al., 1999; Hennekam et al., 2010) In addition, traits and syndromes with autosomal dominant inheritance typically have **varying degrees of severity** in individuals who show any evidence of the condition, which is termed **variable expressivity** of the phenotype. Thus analyzing the genome/genotype of even traits or syndromes with autosomal dominant may not "precisely" predict the phenotype, but certainly can often indicate there will be a major effect on growth and development to some degree. Variable expressivity also may apply to the pleiotropic effect of a particular genotype; that is the expression of a gene resulting in seemingly disparate traits in an individual. Thus even dominant traits that are said to be due to a change in a single gene can be influenced by the proteins from other genes and environmental factors (see figure 2).

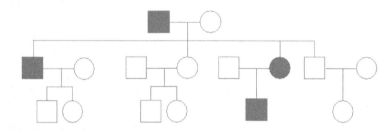

Fig. 1. Autosomal dominant Inheritance.

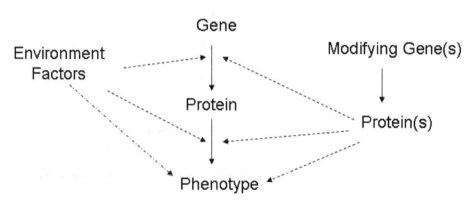

Fig. 2. Interaction of Genetic and Environmental Factors on an "Monogenic Dominant" Trait.

In **autosomal recessive inheritance** the transmission of the pedigree is typically horizontal (present only in siblings, see figure 3). Parents of a child with a trait or syndrome that has an autosomal recessive mode of inheritance are typically heterozygous ("carriers"). The heterozygous parents would then have a 25% of each child of theirs having the autosomal recessive trait or syndrome.

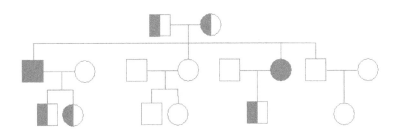

Fig. 3. Autosomal recessive inheritance.

For X linked traits, recessive genes on the one male X chromosome express themselves phenotypically as if they were dominant genes because a male usually only has one X chromosome (hemizygous). In this case the males with the genotype are affected in the pedigree, although in some cases the females can be affected as well. Females who are heterozygous for the gene associated with the X linked recessive phenotype may show some expression of the phenotype. This is because most of the genes on one of the X chromosomes in each cell of a female normally will be inactivated by a process called **lyonization (or X chromosome inactivation)**. Early in fetal development (at approximately the 16-cell morula stage), each cell of the developing female fetus inactivates almost all the genes on one of her two X chromosomes, and all cells that develop from that cell will show the inactivation of the same X chromosome. Depending on the ratio of cells with the X chromosome that has the recessive gene on it versus the X chromosome that does not have the recessive gene, the female may show some variable manifestation of the condition.

Most traits do not adhere to patterns of Mendelian inheritance. These traits are referred to as complex or common diseases and traits, and reflect their complex interaction between genes from more than one locus and environmental factors. Polygenic traits infer the effect of multiple genes on the phenotype, but can be affected by environmental factors also (see figure 4). The distinction between polygenic traits and multifactorial traits (both are traits influenced by environmental and multiple genetic factors) has been made for some multifactorial traits that are discrete (dichotomous) and that occur in an individual once a developmental threshold of genetic and environmental factors to produce the phenotype has been reached.

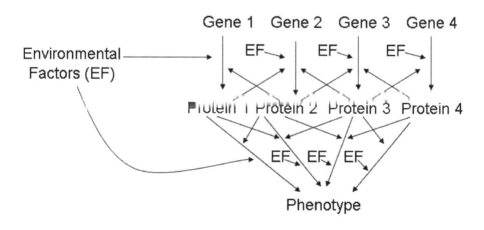

Fig. 4. Interaction of Genetic and Environmental Factors on a Complex Trait.

Epigenetics is the study of acquired and heritable changes in gene function that occur without a change in the DNA sequence. Environmental factors can influence epigenetic mechanisms such as DNA modification (i.e., methylation), histone modification (e.g., lysine and arginine methylation, acetylation, ubiquitination, phosphorylation, sumoylation, ADP ribosylation, deamination and proline isomerization)), and post-transcriptional silencing by RNA interference (microRNA, miRNA). All of these processes can result in gene activation and inactivation.(Lambert & Herceg, 2011) Epigenetic mechanisms can mediate the effect of the environment (e.g., dietary, hormonal and respiratory factors) on the human genome by controlling the transcriptional activity of specific genes, at specific points in time in specific organs.(Gabory et al., 2009; Schwartz, 2010) Malocclusion is a trait than can be greatly influenced by environmental factors. Corrucini suggested that the rapid increase in malocclusion in indigenous Australian people was produced by dietary factors concurrent with industrialization, and emphasized the importance of environmental influences on occlusal variation and the variability of apparent genetic determinants with respect to the environment or population in which they are measured.(Corruccini, 1984, 1990; Corruccini et al., 1990) Likewise Kawala et al. after studying the concordance of malocclusion in twins showed the distribution of within-pair malocclusions depended upon the gender of the individuals, and supported the impact of environmental factors.(Kawala et al., 2007)

In the consideration of environmental effects upon the development of malocclusion, it should not be forgotten that one's genome may influence the response to environmental factors. This is supported by the differences in shape of the mandibular condyles being "slightly greater" among four different inbred strains of mice on a hard diet than on a soft diet for six weeks. When the environment changed sufficiently, the response was different among animals with different genotypes that were not different before the environmental change.(Lavelle, 1983) Siblings may often have similar malocclusions not just because of common genetic or environmental factors, but also because of their shared genetic factors affecting how they respond to the shared environmental factors.(King et al., 1993) However, none of these studies on the effect of environmental factors were focused on epigenetic modifications as a result of environmental factors influencing malocclusion. As the exploration of epigenetics continues throughout biology and medicine, it may also be an interesting area to explore in facial growth.

3. Heritability and malocclusion

Most problems in orthodontics (or any outcome of growth), unless acquired by trauma, are not strictly the result of only genetic or only environmental factors. The ideal occlusion condition shows a proportional growth between the cranial base, the maxilla and the mandible; and involves the harmonious relation between skeletal bases and soft tissues (perioral musculature, lips and tongue).(Mossey, 1999b) The general morphology of craniofacial bones and teeth are largely genetically determined, although clearly variation is partly attributable to environmental factors.(Corruccini et al., 1990; Harris, 2008; Klingenberg et al., 2004; Kraus & Lufkin, 2006; Thesleff, 2006; Townsend et al., 2003) Genetic mechanisms predominate during embryonic craniofacial morphogenesis and in the etiology of many craniofacial abnormalities, therefore genetic factors must be considered in the etiology of malocclusion. However environment is also thought to influence dentofacial morphology postnatally, particularly during facial growth. In response to the presumption of the genome being the predetermining force for facial development and by inference skeletal malocclusion, the Functional Matrix Hypothesis by Moss theorized the primary role of function in craniofacial growth and development. Still, Moss did conclude that both genomic and environmental/epigenetic factors are necessary causes, that neither alone is a sufficient cause and that only the two interacting together furnish both the necessary and sufficient cause(s) of growth and development.(Moss, 1997b, 1997a)

One method employed to estimate this relative contribution of genetic and environmental factors is by calculating the heritability of a trait. Heritability in the broad since (H^2) includes all additive, interactive and other types of genetic and environmental influences. This is impossible to derive, since all the factors and how they interact is not known. Therefore heritability estimates in the literature are in the narrow sense (h^2), and represent the proportion of the total phenotypic variance in a sample that is contributed by additive genetic variance. However, the estimated ratio of genetic variation does not take into account gene-gene or gene-environment interaction.(Hartsfield, 2011) Numerous studies have examined how genetic variation contributes to either or both occlusal and skeletal variation among family members. It is difficult to estimate the influence of environmental (treatment) factors in craniofacial growth because the heritability studies of occlusion are typically based on twins and siblings who did not receive orthodontic treatment. Twin pairs and other groups of siblings containing one or more treated patients (with moderate to severe malocclusion) may have been excluded from most studies. Moreover the twin studies have not included extensive analysis of the parents, nor familial, and nutritional habits; and usually have not compared the twin group with a control group to ascertain environmental covariance (similarity due to twins and other siblings being in a common environment). Therefore, estimates of genetic and environmental contributions may have been affected by lack of accounting for a common environmental effect(Corruccini & Potter, 1980) and ascertainment bias.(King et al., 1993)

The cause of most skeletal- and dentoalveolar based malocclusions is essentially multifactorial in the sense that many diverse causes converge to produce the observed outcome.(King et al., 1993) Numerous studies have examined how genetic variation contributes to either or both occlusal and skeletal variation among family members.(Arya et al., 1973; Boraas et al., 1988; Byard et al., 1985; Cassidy et al., 1998; Chung & Niswander, 1975; Corruccini et al., 1986; Devor, 1987; Ferney et al., 1967, Gass et al. 2003, Harris et al., 1973; Harris et al 1975; Harris & Smith, 1980; Harris & Johnson, 1991; Hauspie et al., 1985; Horowitz et al., 1960; Hunter et al., 1970; Johannsdottir et al., 2005; King et al., 1993; Kraus et al., 1959; Litton et al., 1970; Lobb, 1987; Lundstrom & McWilliam, 1987; Manfredi et al., 1997; Nakata et al., 1973; Nikolova, 1996; Proffit, 1986; Saunders et al., 1980; Susanne & Sharma, 1978; Watnick, 1972) In most studies (particularly those that try to account for bias from the effect of shared environmental factors, unequal means, and unequal variances in monozygotic and dizygotic twin samples),(Harris & Potter, 1997) variations in cephalometric skeletal dimensions are associated in general with a moderate to high degree of genetic variation, whereas in general, variation of occlusal relationships has little or no association with genetic variation.(Harris, 2008)

Although the heritability estimates are low, most of the studies that looked at occlusal traits found that genetic variation is positively correlated with phenotypic variation for arch width and arch length more than for overjet, overbite, and molar relationship. Still, arch size and shape are associated more with environmental variation than with genetic variation.(Cassidy et al., 1998) Because many occlusal variables reflect the combined variations of tooth position and basal and alveolar bone development, these variables (e.g., overjet, overbite, and molar relationship) cannot be less variable than the supporting structures. They will vary because of their own variation in position and those of the basilar structures.(Harris & Johnson, 1991) Heritability studies must be supplemented and to some degree superseded by studies linking or associating specific traits with variation in genetic markers such as single nucleotide polymorphisms (SNPs), variable number of tandem repeats, or other types of specific DNA variation.

For example, SNPs in the EDA gene and the gene for its receptor XEDAR, were found to be associated with dental crowding greater than 5 mm in a Hong Kong Chinese Class I malocclusion sample. It was thought that this may at least be due in part to variation in tooth size as the gene product of EDA is involved in tooth development, and mutations in EDA cause X-linked Hypohydrotic Ectodermal Dysplasia.(Ting et al., 2011) A possible affect on tooth size is consistent with the findings that in skeletal Class I crowding cases tooth size variation may more often play a role than skeletal growth.(Bernabe & Flores-Mir, 2006; Hashim & Al-Ghamdi, 2005; Poosti & Jalali, 2007; Ting et al., 2011) Although these genes are located on the X chromosome, the associations remained after adjustment for sex. This type of investigation is thought to help get around the problem of confounding environmental factors, although an increased analysis of epigenetic markers may show this is not that simple. Still these studies are the only way in which possible predictive data will be collected and tested.

4. Use of family data to predict growth

Siblings have been noted as often showing similar types of malocclusion. Examination of parents and older siblings has been suggested as a way to gain information regarding the treatment need for a child, including early treatment of malocclusion.(Harris & Kowalski, 1976; Litton et al., 1970; Niswander, 1975; Saunders et al., 1980) Niswander noted that the frequency of malocclusion is decreased among siblings of index cases with normal occlusion, whereas the siblings of index cases with malocclusion tend to have the same type of malocclusion more often. (Niswander, 1975) There are high correlation coefficient values between parents and their offspring for Class II and Class III malocclusions.(Nakasima et al., 1982) It has been shown that the craniofacial skeletal patterns of children with Class II (division 1) malocclusions are familial (i.e., occur more often in multiple members of some families), and that a high resemblance to the skeletal patterns occurs in their siblings with normal occlusion.(Harris et al., 1975) Although this was ascribed to the Class II (division 1) being "heritable," common environmental factors were not taken into account. From this it was concluded that the genetic basis for this resemblance is probably polygenic, and family skeletal patterns were used as predictors for the treatment prognosis of the child with a Class II malocclusion, although it was acknowledged that the current morphology of the patient is the primary source of information about future growth.(Harris & Kowalski, 1976)

Each child receives half of his or her genes from each parent, but not likely the same combination of genes as a sibling unless the children are monozygotic twins. When looking at parents with a differing skeletal morphology, knowing which of the genes in what combination from each parent is present in the child is difficult until the child's phenotype matures under the continuing influence of environmental factors. When considering polygenic traits, the highest phenotypic correlation that can be expected based on genes in common by inheritance from one parent to a child, or between siblings, is 0.5. Because the child's phenotype is likely to be influenced by the interaction of genes from both parents, the "mid-parent" value may increase the correlation with their children to 0.7 because of the regression to the mean of parental dimensions in their children. Squaring the correlation between the two variables derives the amount of variation predicted for one variable in correlation with another variable. Therefore, at best, using mid-parent values, only 49% of the variability of any facial dimension in a child can be predicted by consideration of the average of the same dimension in the parents. Only 25% of the variability of any facial dimension in a child can be predicted, at best, by considering the same dimension in a sibling or one parent. Because varying effects of environmental factors interact with the multiple genetic factors, the usual correlation for facial dimensions between parents and their children is about 30%, yielding even less predictive power.(Hunter, 1990)

In most patients, the mode of inheritance for the craniofacial skeleton is polygenic (complex). However, in some families (e.g., with a relatively prognathic mandible compared with the maxilla), the mode of inheritance is not polygenic. Future research may investigate the genetic factors that do not fit a polygenic mode that may be present in some families. Identification of those factors will increase the ability to predict the likelihood of a particular resulting morphology. Unfortunately, orthodontists do not have sufficient information to make accurate predictions about the development of occlusion simply by studying the frequency of its occurrence in parents or even siblings. Admittedly, family patterns of resemblance are frequently obvious, and observed family tendencies should not be ignored.

Nonetheless, predictions must be made cautiously because genetic and environmental factors and their interaction are unknown and difficult to evaluate and predict with precision.(Hartsfield, 2011)

5. Genetic markers associated with variations in growth of complex etiology

5.1 Growth hormone receptor

Growth hormone is an important factor in craniofacial and skeletal growth. A variant in the growth hormone receptor and its gene (GHR), when there is a proline amino acid instead of threonine at the 561st residue in the protein, is referred to as the GHR P56IT allele. Of a normal Japanese sample of 50 men and 50 women, those who did not have the GHR P56IT allele had a significantly greater mandibular ramus length (condylion-gonion) than did those with the GHR P56IT allele. The average mandibular ramus height in those with the GHR P56IT allele was 4.65 mm shorter than the average for those without the GHR P56IT allele. This significant correlation between the GHR P56IT allele and shorter mandibular ramus height was confirmed in an additional 80 women.(Yamaguchi et al., 2001) Interestingly, the association was with the mandibular ramus height but not mandibular body length, maxillary length, or anterior cranial base length. This suggests a site-, area-, or region-specific effect. The study concluded that the GHR P56IT allele may be associated with mandibular height growth and can be a genetic marker for it. Still, whether the effect is directly on the mandible or some other nearby tissue or on another matrix is not clear. It has been suggested that GHR variants P561T and C422F are associated with mandibular ramus height in Japanese population and that the SNPs of the GHR gene associated with differences in mandibular ramus height in the Japanese are likely to be different in other ethnic groups. (Tomoyasu et al., 2009)

This is supported by the finding that although there is a possible association between the GHR polymorphisms P561T, C422F and "haplotype 4" in a Korean population, there was not significant association between these markers and mandibular height in African-Americans, European-Americans, and Hispanics.(Kang et al., 2009) This group suggested that this finding might partly explain the differing craniofacial morphology among different ethnicities. Analysis of the possible association between the P561T variant in the GHR gene and mandibular growth during early childhood did not find a difference between mandibular protrusion and normal occlusion. (Sasaki et al., 2009) To see what effect different diets would have on individuals with and without the GHR P56IT allele would be interesting as a means of looking at genetic and environmental factor interaction. Undoubtedly many other genes that may influence craniofacial structure, including ramus height, could be identified, and their variation could be studied along with different environmental factors (e.g., orthodontic treatment) and the resulting phenotype.

5.2 Growth differences during puberty

Increased accuracy in the estimation of pubertal facial growth would be of great benefit prior to the utilization of different therapeutic modalities including orthodontics, orthopedic growth modification and surgery. Research and discussion about facial growth and treatment in the literature have focused either on the timing of the greatest amount of facial growth, particularly for the mandible(Gu & McNamara, 2007; Hunter et al., 2007; Verma et al., 2009); or the estimated extent of facial growth to be attained.(Chvatal et al., 2005; Turchetta et al., 2007) As useful as average facial growth predictions based upon expected growth curves may be, more valid prediction must incorporate and account for the variation associated with individual genetic factors, particularly those that are highly pertinent to the pubertal growth spurt. The pubertal growth spurt response is mediated by the combination of sex steroids, growth hormone, insulin-like growth factor (IGF-I) and other endocrine, paracrine and autocrine factors. Testosterone and estradiol in mice have a direct, sex-specific stimulatory activity on male and female derived chondroprogenitor cell proliferation. Testosterone stimulated growth and local production of IGF-I and IGF-I-R in chondrocyte cell layers of an isolated organ culture of mice mandibular condyle.(Maor et al., 1999) Investigation into the effects of neonatal surgical castration and prepubertal chemical castration on craniofacial growth in rats showed that craniofacial growth was related to testosterone concentration. Administration of low doses of testosterone in boys with delayed puberty not only accelerates their statural growth rate, but their craniofacial growth rate as well.(Verdonck et al., 1998; Verdonck et al., 1999)

Ovariectomized and orchiectomized mice that sex hormone levels influenced condylar morphogenesis changed the internal structure of the mandibular condyle.(Fujita et al., 2001) It has been suggested that the suppression of sex hormone secretion in the growth phase might inhibit craniofacial growth and result in poor craniofacial development, particularly nasomaxillary bone and mandible, in new born and pubertal rats.(Fujita et al., 2004; Fujita et al., 2006) It has been demonstrated using administration of sex hormone specific receptor antagonists that growth of the mandible and femur is induced in response to the stimulation of the estrogen receptor beta (ERβ) in chondrocytes before and during early puberty in mice. In late and after puberty, the growth is induced by the stimulation of estrogen receptor alpha (ERα) in male and female mice. From this it was proposed that a screen of sex hormones could be used as an indicator of bone maturity to accurately predict the beginning and end of growth in orthodontic treatment.

CYP19A1 is the gene that encodes aromatase. This enzyme catalyzes the rate limiting step in estrogen biosynthesis by converting androgens. In order to best diagnose and treat the child or adolescent patient, the orthodontist needs to know as much as possible about the patient's growth potential. As useful as predictions based upon expected growth models starting from early in the patient's life may be, prediction must incorporate and account for the variation associated with individual genetic factors, especially those that are highly pertinent to the pubertal growth spurt.

Estrogens are a group of hormones involved in growth and development.(Honjo et al., 1992) Estrogen stimulates chondrogenesis, promotes the progressive closure of the epiphyseal growth plate, has an anabolic effect on the osteoblast and an apoptotic effect on the osteoclast, and increases bone mineral acquisition in axial and appendicular bone during adolescence and into the third decade.(Grumbach, 2000) Aromatase (also known as estrogen synthetase) is a key cytochrome P450 enzyme involved in estrogen biosynthesis.(Bulun et al., 2003) This steroidogenic enzyme catalyzes the final step of estrogen biosynthesis by converting testosterone and androstenedione to estradiol and estrone, respectively.(Guo et al., 2006) Regulation of this gene's transcription is critical for the testosterone/estrogen (T/E) ratio in the body since aromatase plays an important role in the conversion of androgens to estrogens. Some studies have shown that the T/E ratio is critical in the development of sex-indexed facial characteristics such as the growth of cheekbones, the mandible and chin, the prominence of eyebrow ridges and the lengthening of the lower face. (Schaefer et al., 2005; Schaefer et al., 2006)

The difference in the average sagittal jaw growth between the two groups of Caucasian males with different *CYP19A1* alleles with the greatest differences in growth per year was just over 1.5 mm per year during treatment for the maxilla, and 2.5 mm per year for the mandible. (Hartsfield Jr. et al., 2010) There was no statistical difference for the particular *CYP19A1* alleles in females. This is particularly impressive since at the beginning of treatment there was no significant difference among the males based upon the *CYP19A1* genotype. The significant difference only expressed itself over the time of treatment during the cervical vertebral stage associated with increased growth velocity.(Hartsfield et al., 2010) Interestingly the same result was found in a group of Chinese males and females, strongly suggesting that this variation in the *CYP19A1* gene may be a multi-ethnic marker for sagittal facial growth. (He et al., 2011) Although the difference in average annual sagittal mandibular and maxillary growth based upon this *CYP19A1* genotype were significant, as one factor in a complex trait (sagittal jaw growth), they account for only part of the variation seen, and therefore by itself has little predictive power. Further investigation of this and other genetic factors, their interactions with each other and with environmental factors will help to explain what has up to now been an unknown component of individual variations in facial growth.

5.3 Class II division 2 (Class II/2) malocclusion

There is evidence that Class II division 2, and particularly Class III malocclusions, can have a strong genetic component. The Class II division 2 (II/2) malocclusion is a relatively rare type of malocclusion, representing between 2.3% and 5% of all malocclusions in the western white population.(Ast et al., 1965; Mills, 1966) In one study 100% of 20 monozygotic (MZ) twin pairs were concordant for II/2 malocclusion, while only 10.7% of 28 dizygotic (DZ) twin pairs demonstrated concordance for the Class II/2 malocclusion. (Markovic, 1992) These findings suggest the effect of common genetic or environmental factors; however, the much lower concordance for DZ twins would suggest that multiple genetic factors rather than a single gene contribute to the risk for Class II/2. This was reinforced by Ruf et al. concluding that the etiology of Class II/2 malocclusion was unclear, with neither form nor function the sole controlling factor.(Ruf & Pancherz, 1999)

From a developmental viewpoint it is interesting that there is a strong association of Class II/2 malocclusion with dental developmental anomalies, more so than for other Angle malocclusion classes.(Basdra et al., 2001) Excluding 3rd molars, agenesis of other teeth was at least three times more common in Class II/2 subjects than in the general population. In addition, there were a significantly greater number of dental developmental anomalies present in Class II/2 subjects as compared to the general population. They found 56.6% of Class II/2 patients exhibited developmental tooth anomalies including hypodontia as compared to as many as 35% of the general population having agenesis of one or more third molar.(Basdra et al., 2000) In addition Peck et al. showed a statistically significant reduction in permanent maxillary incisor mesial-distal width associated with Class II/2.(Peck et al., 1998)

Further evidence for a polygenic complex etiology for Class II/2 was found in a study of 68 subjects (67 self reported as white and 1 white/African-American who was a child of one of the 18 probands). (Morrison, 2008) A proband is the affected individual through whom a family is first seen or studied for a genetic trait, syndrome or disorder. In this study, researchers included 50 reported first-degree relatives of each proband, with a minimum of 2 first-degree relatives of each proband. The findings showed a marked increase in the number of females affected with Class II/2 in both the probands and their first-degree relatives than affected males. Of the 36 first-degree relatives whose occlusion was analyzed, 6 (16.7%) were found to be Class II/2. The relative risk (RR) of first-degree relatives to have a Class II/2 was found to be 3.3 – 7.3. The confidence interval (CI) was 1.1-10.3 if the RR was 3.3 and 1.7-31.6 if the RR was 7.3.

Agenesis of one or more permanent teeth (excluding 3rd molars) was found in 2 (11.1%) of the 18 probands and 7 (14.0%) of the 50 first-degree relatives. Agenesis of one or more 3rd molars was found in 4 (22.2%) of the 18 probands and 12 (24.0%) of the 50 first-degree relatives. Agenesis of one or both permanent maxillary incisors was found in none of the 18 probands and 2 (4.0%) of the 50 first-degree relatives. One or more small teeth (excluding 3rd molars) were found in 4 (22.2%) of the 18 probands and 15 (30.0%) of the 50 first-degree relatives. Small maxillary permanent incisors were found in none of the 18 probands and 4 (8.0%) of the 50 first-degree relatives. Agenesis of one or more permanent teeth in combination with the presence of one or more small permanent teeth was found in 2 (11.1%) of the 18 probands and 7 (14.0%) of the 50 first-degree relatives. Of the 36 first-degree relatives evaluated for malocclusion, 6 (16.67%) were found to be Class II/2. The RR for first-degree relatives of the probands to have a Class II/2 malocclusion was 3.3 – 7.35.(Morrison, 2008)

These results indicate that first-degree relatives of Class II/2 probands have a significantly increased risk of having a Class II/2 malocclusion as compared with individuals from the general population. Were Class II/2 malocclusion to be the result of variation in a single gene, acting in either a dominant or recessive fashion, the relative risk would be expected to be much higher. Rather, the modest, albeit significant increase in risk appears consistent with results from previous studies, which suggest a multifactorial etiology for Class II/2 malocclusion.

The question could be raised as to whether or not anomalous maxillary lateral incisors are associated with the Class II/2 malocclusion phenotype, and therefore share common etiological factors. Basdra et al. showed that 13.9% of Class II/2 subjects had agenesis of maxillary lateral incisors and 7.5% had peg-shaped or small maxillary lateral incisors. In contrast, Morrison found none of the probands had agenesis of or small maxillary lateral incisors, although first-degree relatives of the Class II/2 probands showed similar frequencies of hypodontia and microdontia of other teeth as the II/2 probands. However, the frequencies of these dental anomalies in the probands and first degree relatives were not significantly greater than those in the general population.(Morrison, 2008) Thus it is unclear if Class II/2 probands and their first-degree relatives are at an increased risk of developing hypodontia and/or microdontia. Investigations of a larger sample of Class II/2 subjects and relatives to address that question and possible common etiological factors, including genes associated with tooth development and hypodontia, are needed.

A start on this was made when DNA markers (single nucleotide polymorphisms, also referred to as SNPs) in two genes associated with dental development and or hypodontia, *MSX1*, *PAX9, AXIN2*. *RUNX2* and *RUNX3* were investigated in 94 Class II/2 Caucasian subjects (31 with hypodontia) compared to 89 non-Class II/2 Caucasian subjects without hypodontia. (Morford et al., 2010b; Morford et al., 2010a) A borderline-association of all Class II/2 subjects with the *PAX9* SNP (rs8004560) was identified (p=0.06). A borderline-association of the same rs8004560 *PAX9* SNP was also identified for subjects with Class II/2 with hypodontia of any permanent tooth, excluding third-molars, when compared to non-Class II/2 without hypodontia (p=0.08) but not when compared to Class II/2 without hypodontia (p=0.46). No associations of Class II/2 with the *PAX9* rs1955734, *MSX1* rs3821949, *RUNX2* (rs1406846), *RUNX3* (rs6672420), or *AXIN2* (rs7591, rs2240308) genotypes were identified. There was a significant association (p=0.0284) for Class II/2 subjects (with or without hypodontia) and the *RUNX2* rs6930053 SNP. However, there was no association of *RUNX2* rs6930053 for subjects with Class II/2 that had hypodontia of any permanent tooth, including third-molars, when compared to Class II/2 subjects without hypodontia (p=0.3858). This suggests a mild impact of *PAX9* (or a locus in linkage-disequilibrium with it) on the development of Class II/2 with hypodontia, and that *RUNX2* (or genetic loci in linkage-disequilibrium with *RUNX2*) plays a role in Class II/2 development but not in the occasionally-associated hypodontia. These findings and other DNA markers should be investigated in a larger Caucasian and other ethnic groups.(Malinowski, 1983; Strohmayer, 1937; Suzuki, 1961)

5.4 Class III malocclusion

Although all Angle occlusion types a Class III malocclusion were initially only based on the sagittal relationship of the permanent first molars, it has generally been recognized that this dental relationship is often observed with a corresponding skeletal relationship as well. Thus, the Class III malocclusion is a complex disorder characterized by a combination of dental and skeletal features that characteristically result in the appearance of a prominent lower jaw. Often referred to as mandibular prognathism (taken from the Greek pro =forward and gnathos =jaw), skeletal aspects of this disorder can be a result of pure mandibular prognathism, maxillary hypoplasia/retrognathism, or a combination of the two. These phenotypic variations create a significant heterogeneity among Class III subjects that can vary according to sex and ethnicity, and account for some of the difficulty encountered when investigating the condition.(Singh, 1999) The familial nature of mandibular prognathism was first reported by Strohmayer (1937) as noted by Wolff et al (1993) in their analysis of the pedigree of the Hapsburg family.(Wolff et al., 1993)

The highest prevalence of Class III malocclusion is observed in East Asian populations such as Korean, Chinese, and Japanese (8%-40%).(Allwright, 1964; Ishii et al., 2002) By comparison, African populations exhibit a reduced prevalence rate (3-8%) compared to Asian samples(Emrich et al., 1965; Garner & Butt, 1985), as do individuals of European or European-American (Caucasian) decent (reports varying between 0.48%-9.5%, with most in the 3-5% range)(Davidov et al., 1961; Emrich et al., 1965; Goose et al., 1957; Helm, 1968; Horowitz, 1970; Ingervall, 1974; Laine & Hausen, 1983; Luffingham & Campbell, 1974; Massler & Frankel, 1951; Solow & Helm, 1968; Tipton & Rinchuse, 1991) While the prevalence in a sample of Native American Chippewa Indian children is relatively low (2.6-3.1%),(Grewe et al., 1968) North American Eskimos in Labrador, Canada have a class III prevalence of approximately 16%.(Zammit et al., 1995) (Zammit, Hans, et al. 1995)

Populations in South America are often a mixture of Caucasian/European, African and Amerindian decent. While the percentage of children in Bogotá, Colombia with Class III has been reported as 3.7%, Brazilian children exhibited a frequency between 4 -10%.(Grando et al., 2008; Martins Mda & Lima, 2009; Thilander et al., 2001) In areas of the Middle East, the prevalence of class III also displays variation with the highest prevalence in Egypt at 10.6%,(El-Mangoury & Mostafa, 1990) followed by 7.8% in Iran,(Borzabadi-Farahani et al., 2009) and 5.1% in Lebanon.(Saleh, 1999)

Several studies have suggested the existence of multiple patterns or sub-phenotypes of the Class III malocclusion based on anatomical appearance. For example, Ellis and McNamara reported considerable variation among class III patients. The most common combination of variables was a retrusive maxilla, protrusive maxillary incisors, retrusive mandibular incisors, a protrusive mandible, and a long lower facial height.(Ellis & McNamara, 1984) Although they did not find significant sex differences, Baccetti et al. showed a significant degree of sexual dimorphism in craniofacial features in subjects with class III malocclusion.(Baccetti et al., 2005) The female Class III subjects presented smaller linear dimensions in the maxilla, mandible, and anterior facial heights when compared with male subjects. The increase in mandibular growth was three times greater in males with class III than in subjects with normal occlusion.(Baccetti et al., 2007) Martone and colleagues suggested that craniofacial growth generates several head form types resulting in anatomic sub-groupings of Classes III.(Martone et al., 1992) Mackay et al (1992) identified five Class III subgroups, all of which exhibited mandibular prognathism.(Mackay et al., 1992) English children with Class III malocclusions divided into groups (normal anteroposterior positioned mandibles and protruded mandibles) according to their SNB angle were found to have significant differences in both groups relating to sagittal position of the maxilla and mandibular rotation.(Hashim & Sarhan, 1993)

Bui et al (2006) found five clusters representing distinct subphenotypes of class III malocclusion. The groupings of variables reflected anteroposterior and vertical dimensions rather than specific craniofacial structures, suggesting that different genes are involved in controlling dimension versus structure. The five subgroupings or "Prototype Clusters" were described as follows: (1) prognathic mandible with long face, (2) maxillary deficiency with decreased vertical dimension (low angle), (3) maxillary deficiency with increased vertical dimension (high angle), (4) mild prognathic mandible with normal vertical dimension, and (5) a combination of prognathic mandible and maxillary deficiency with normal vertical dimension.(Bui et al., 2006) Further studies of the variation of the subtypes of the Class III phenotype within families should facilitate increased understanding of the genetic and non-genetic factors involved.

The genetic factors appear to be heterogeneous, with monogenic (usually autosomal dominant with incomplete penetrance and variable expressivity) influences in some families and multifactorial (polygenic complex) influences in others.(Cruz et al., 2008; Downs, 1927 ; El-Gheriani et al., 2003; Krauss et al., 1959; Litton et al., 1970; Niswander, 1975; Stiles & Luke, 1953; Strohmayer, 1937; Thompson & Winter, 1988; Wolff et al., 1993) This contributes to the variety of anatomical changes in the cranial base, maxilla, and mandible that may be associated with "mandibular prognathism" or a Class III malocclusion.(Bui et al., 2006; Singh, 1999) The prevalence of Class III malocclusion varies among races and can show different anatomic characteristics between races.(Ishii et al., 2002) Considering this heterogeneity, and possible epistasis (the interaction between or among gene products on their expression) and even epigenetics, it is not surprising that genetic linkage and candidate gene studies to date have indicated the possible location of genetic loci influencing this trait in several chromosomal locations (see figure 5).(Falcão-Alencar et al., 2010; Frazier-Bowers et al., 2009; Jang et al., 2010; Li et al., 2010; Li et al., 2011; Tassopoulou-Fishell et al., 2011; Xue et al., 2010; Yamaguchi et al., 2005)

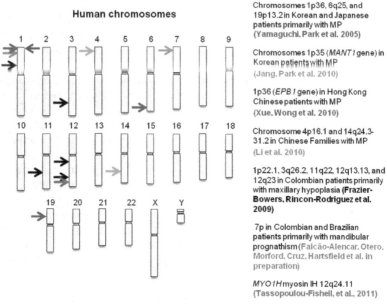

Human chromosomes

Chromosomes 1p36, 6q25, and 19p13.2 in Korean and Japanese patients primarily with MP (Yamaguchi, Park et al. 2005)

Chromosomes 1p35 (*MANT1* gene) in Korean patients with MP (Jang, Park et al. 2010)

1p36 (*EPB1* gene) in Hong Kong Chinese patients with MP (Xue, Wong et al. 2010)

Chromosome 4p16.1 and 14q24.3-31.2 in Chinese Families with MP (Li et al. 2010)

1p22.1, 3q26.2, 11q22, 12q13.13, and 12q23 in Colombian patients primarily with maxillary hypoplasia **(Frazier-Bowers, Rincon-Rodriguez et al. 2009)**

7p in Colombian and Brazilian patients primarily with mandibular prognathism (Falcão-Alencar, Otero, Morford, Cruz, Hartsfield et al. in preparation)

MYO1H myosin IH 12q24.11 (Tassopoulou-Fishell, et al., 2011)

Fig. 5. Chromosome location of markers linked or associated with Class III malocclusion in humans.

6. Personalized orthdontics

In summary, "Personalized Medicine" is a new buzz phrase, based initially upon pharmacogenetics and now exploding as genome-wide association and pathway studies are undertaken. The understanding of the combination and interaction of genetic and environmental (including treatment) factors (nature and nurture together) that influence the growth treatment response of our patients is fundamental to the evidence based practice of orthodontics. Conclusions from retrospective studies must be evaluated by prospective testing to truly evaluate their value in practice. Genome-wide association studies, metabolic pathway analysis and candidate gene studies are necessary to further the evidence base for the practice of orthodontics to determine what the best treatment plan is for each patient in the era of truly personalized orthodontics.(Hartsfield, 2008)

7. References

Allwright, W.C. (1964). A survey of handicapping dentofacial anomalies among Chinese in Hong Kong. *Int Dent J*, Vol. 14, No. 1964), pp. 505-519,

Arya, B.S., Savara, B.S., Clarkson, Q.D. & Thomas, D.R. (1973). Genetic variability of craniofacial dimensions. *The Angle orthodontist,* Vol. 43, No. 2, (Apr 1973), pp. 207-215, 0003-3219 (Print)

Ast, D.B., Carlos, J.P. & Cons, N.C. (1965). The Prevalence and Characteristics of Malocclusion among Senior High School Students in Upstate New York. *American journal of orthodontics,* Vol. 51, No. (Jun 1965), pp. 437-445, 0002-9416

Baccetti, T., Reyes, B.C. & McNamara, J.A., Jr. (2005). Gender differences in Class III malocclusion. *The Angle orthodontist,* Vol. 75, No. 4, (Jul 2005), pp. 510-520, 0003-3219 (Print) 0003-3219 (Linking)

Baccetti, T., Reyes, B.C. & McNamara, J.A., Jr. (2007). Craniofacial changes in Class III malocclusion as related to skeletal and dental maturation. *American journal of orthodontics and dentofacial orthopedics : official publication of the American Association of Orthodontists, its constituent societies, and the American Board of Orthodontics,* Vol. 132, No. 2, (Aug 2007), pp. 171 e171-171 e112, 1097-6752 (Electronic) 0889-5406 (Linking)

Basdra, E.K., Kiokpasoglou, M. & Stellzig, A. (2000). The Class II Division 2 craniofacial type is associated with numerous congenital tooth anomalies. *European journal of orthodontics,* Vol. 22, No. 5, (Oct 2000), pp. 529-535, 0141-5387

Basdra, E.K., Kiokpasoglou, M.N. & Komposch, G. (2001). Congenital tooth anomalies and malocclusions: a genetic link? *European journal of orthodontics,* Vol. 23, No. 2, (Apr 2001), pp. 145-151, 0141-5387

Bernabe, E. & Flores-Mir, C. (2006). Dental morphology and crowding. A multivariate approach. *The Angle orthodontist,* Vol. 76, No. 1, (Jan 2006), pp. 20-25, 0003-3219 (Print) 0003-3219 (Linking)

Boraas, J.C., Messer, L.B. & Till, M.J. (1988). A genetic contribution to dental caries, occlusion, and morphology as demonstrated by twins reared apart. *Journal of dental research,* Vol. 67, No. 9, (Sep 1988), pp. 1150-1155, 0022-0345 (Print)

Borzabadi-Farahani, A., Borzabadi-Farahani, A. & Eslamipour, F. (2009). Malocclusion and occlusal traits in an urban Iranian population. An epidemiological study of 11- to 14-year-old children. *European journal of orthodontics,* Vol. 31, No. 5, (Oct 2009), pp. 477-484, 1460-2210 (Electronic) 0141-5387 (Linking)

Bui, C., King, T., Proffit, W. & Frazier-Bowers, S. (2006). Phenotypic characterization of Class III patients. *The Angle orthodontist,* Vol. 76, No. 4, (Jul 2006), pp. 564-569, 0003-3219 (Print) 0003-3219 (Linking)

Bulun, S.E., Sebastian, S., Takayama, K., Suzuki, T., Sasano, H. & Shozu, M. (2003). The human CYP19 (aromatase P450) gene: update on physiologic roles and genomic organization of promoters. *J Steroid Biochem Mol Biol,* Vol. 86, No. 3-5, (Sep 2003), pp. 219-224, 0960-0760 (Print)

Buschang, P.H. & Hinton, R.J. (2005). A Gradient of Potential for Modifying Craniofacial Growth. *Semin Orthod,* Vol. 11, No. 2005), pp. 219-226,

Byard, P.J., Poosha, D.V., Satyanarayana, M. & Rao, D.C. (1985). Family resemblance for components of craniofacial size and shape. *Journal of craniofacial genetics and developmental biology,* Vol. 5, No. 3, 1985), pp. 229-238, 0270-4145 (Print) 0270-4145 (Linking)

Cassidy, K.M., Harris, E.F., Tolley, E.A. & Keim, R.G. (1998). Genetic influence on dental arch form in orthodontic patients. *The Angle orthodontist,* Vol. 68, No. 5, (Oct 1998), pp. 445-454, 0003-3219 (Print)

Chung, C.S. & Niswander, J.D. (1975). Genetic and epidemiologic studies of oral characteristics in Hawaii's schoolchildren: V. Sibling correlations in occlusion traits. *Journal of dental research,* Vol. 54, No. 2, (Mar-Apr 1975), pp. 324-329, 0022-0345 (Print)

Chvatal, B.A., Behrents, R.G., Ceen, R.F. & Buschang, P.H. (2005). Development and testing of multilevel models for longitudinal craniofacial growth prediction. *American journal of orthodontics and dentofacial orthopedics : official publication of the American Association of Orthodontists, its constituent societies, and the American Board of Orthodontics,* Vol. 128, No. 1, (Jul 2005), pp. 45-56, 0889-5406 (Print)

Corruccini, R.S. & Potter, R.H. (1980). Genetic analysis of occlusal variation in twins. *American journal of orthodontics,* Vol. 78, No. 2, (Aug 1980), pp. 140-154, 0002-9416 (Print)

Corruccini, R.S. (1984). An epidemiologic transition in dental occlusion in world populations. *American journal of orthodontics,* Vol. 86, No. 5, (Nov 1984), pp. 419-426, 0002-9416 (Print)

Corruccini, R.S., Sharma, K. & Potter, R.H. (1986). Comparative genetic variance and heritability of dental occlusal variables in U.S. and Northwest Indian twins. *American journal of physical anthropology,* Vol. 70, No. 3, (Jul 1986), pp. 293-299, 0002-9483 (Print)

Corruccini, R.S. (1990). Australian aboriginal tooth succession, interproximal attrition, and Begg's theory. *American journal of orthodontics and dentofacial orthopedics : official publication of the American Association of Orthodontists, its constituent societies, and the American Board of Orthodontics,* Vol. 97, No. 4, (Apr 1990), pp. 349-357, 0889-5406 (Print) 0889-5406 (Linking)

Corruccini, R.S., Townsend, G.C., Richards, L.C. & Brown, T. (1990). Genetic and environmental determinants of dental occlusal variation in twins of different nationalities. *Hum Biol,* Vol. 62, No. 3, 1990), pp. 353-367.,

Cruz, R.M., Krieger, H., Ferreira, R., Mah, J., Hartsfield, J., Jr. & Oliveira, S. (2008). Major gene and multifactorial inheritance of mandibular prognathism. *American journal of medical genetics. Part A,* Vol. 146A, No. 1, (Jan 1 2008), pp. 71-77, 1552-4833 (Electronic) 1552-4825 (Linking)

Davidov, S., Geseva, N., Donveca, T. & Dehova, L. (1961). Incidence of prognathism in Bulgaria. *Dental Abstracts,* Vol. 6, No. 1961), pp. 240,

Devor, E.J. (1987). Transmission of human craniofacial dimensions. *Journal of craniofacial genetics and developmental biology,* Vol. 7, No. 2, 1987), pp. 95-106, 0270-4145 (Print)

Downs, W.G. (1927). Studies in the Causes of Dental Anomalies. . *Genetics* Vol. 12, No. 6, (Nov 1927 1927), pp. 570-580, 0016-6731 (Print) 0016-6731 (Linking)

El-Gheriani, A.A., Maher, B.S., El-Gheriani, A.S., Sciote, J.J., Abu-Shahba, F.A., Al-Azemi, R. & Marazita, M.L. (2003). Segregation analysis of mandibular prognathism in Libya. *Journal of dental research,* Vol. 82, No. 7, (Jul 2003), pp. 523-527, 0022-0345 (Print) 0022-0345 (Linking)

El-Mangoury, N.H. & Mostafa, Y.A. (1990). Epidemiologic panorama of dental occlusion. *The Angle orthodontist*, Vol. 60, No. 3, (Fall 1990), pp. 207-214, 0003-3219 (Print) 0003-3219 (Linking)

Ellis, E., 3rd & McNamara, J.A., Jr. (1984). Components of adult Class III malocclusion. *J Oral Maxillofacial Surg*, Vol. 42, No. 5, (May 1984), pp. 295-305, 0278-2391 (Print) 0278-2391 (Linking)

Emrich, R.E., Brodie, A.G. & Blayney, J.R. (1965). Prevalence of Class 1, Class 2, and Class 3 malocclusions (Angle) in an urban population. An epidemiological study. *Journal of dental research*, Vol. 44, No. 5, (Sep-Oct 1965), pp. 947-953, 0022-0345 (Print) 0022-0345 (Linking)

Everett, E.T., Britto, D.A., Ward, R.E. & Hartsfield, J.K., Jr. (1999). A novel FGFR2 gene mutation in Crouzon syndrome associated with apparent nonpenetrance. *The Cleft palate-craniofacial journal : official publication of the American Cleft Palate-Craniofacial Association*, Vol. 36, No. 6, (Nov 1999), pp. 533-541, 1055-6656 (Print)

Falcão-Alencar, G., Ortero, L., Cruz, R.M., Foroud, T.M., Dongbing, L., Koller, D., Morford, L.A., Ferrari, I., Oliveira, S.F. & Hartsfield, J.K. (2010). *Evidence for Genetic Linkage of the Class III Craniofacial Phenotype With Human Chromosome 7 in 36 South American Families*, (abstract/program #975). Presented at the 60th Annual Meeting of The American Society of Human Genetics, November 3, 2010, Washington, DC).

Fernex, E., Hauenstein, P. & Roche, M. (1967). [Heredity and craniofacial morphology]. *Report of the congress. European Orthodontic Society*, Vol. No. 1967), pp. 239-257,

Frazier-Bowers, S., Rincon-Rodriguez, R., Zhou, J., Alexander, K. & Lange, E. (2009). Evidence of linkage in a Hispanic cohort with a Class III dentofacial phenotype. *Journal of dental research*, Vol. 88, No. 1, (Jan 2009), pp. 56-60, 1544-0591 (Electronic) 0022-0345 (Linking)

Fujita, T., Kawata, T., Tokimasa, C., Kohno, S., Kaku, M. & Tanne, K. (2001). Breadth of the mandibular condyle affected by disturbances of the sex hormones in ovariectomized and orchiectomized mice. *Clinical orthodontics and research*, Vol. 4, No. 3, (Aug 2001), pp. 172-176, 1397-5927 (Print) 1397-5927 (Linking)

Fujita, T., Ohtani, J., Shigekawa, M., Kawata, T., Kaku, M., Kohno, S., Tsutsui, K., Tenjo, K., Motokawa, M., Tohma, Y. & Tanne, K. (2004). Effects of sex hormone disturbances on craniofacial growth in newborn mice. *Journal of dental research*, Vol. 83, No. 3, (Mar 2004), pp. 250-254, 0022-0345 (Print) 0022-0345 (Linking)

Fujita, T., Ohtani, J., Shigekawa, M., Kawata, T., Kaku, M., Kohno, S., Motokawa, M., Tohma, Y. & Tanne, K. (2006). Influence of sex hormone disturbances on the internal structure of the mandible in newborn mice. *European journal of orthodontics*, Vol. 28, No. 2, (Apr 2006), pp. 190-194, 0141-5387 (Print) 0141-5387 (Linking)

Gabory, A., Attig, L. & Junien, C. (2009). Sexual dimorphism in environmental epigenetic programming. *Molecular and cellular endocrinology*, Vol. 304, No. 1-2, (May 25 2009), pp. 8-18, 1872-8057 (Electronic) 0303-7207 (Linking)

Garner, L.D. & Butt, M.H. (1985). Malocclusion in black Americans and Nyeri Kenyans. An epidemiologic study. *The Angle orthodontist,* Vol. 55, No. 2, (Apr 1985), pp. 139-146, 0003-3219 (Print) 0003-3219 (Linking)

Gass, J.R., Valiathan, M., Tiwari, H.K., Hans, M.G. & Elston, R.C. (2003). Familial correlations and heritability of maxillary midline diastema. *American journal of orthodontics and dentofacial orthopedics : official publication of the American Association of Orthodontists, its constituent societies, and the American Board of Orthodontics,* Vol. 123, No. 1, (Jan 2003), pp. 35-39, 0889-5406 (Print)

Goose, D.H., Thomson, D.G. & Winter, F.C. (1957). Malocclusion in schoolchildren of the west Midlands. *British Dental Journal,* Vol. 102, No. 1957), pp. 174-178,

Grando, C., Young, A.A., Vedovello Filho, M., Vedovello, S.A. & Ramirez-Yanez, G.O. (2008). Prevalence of malocclusions in a young Brazilian population. *International journal of orthodontics,* Vol. 19, No. 2, (Summer 2008), pp. 13-16, 1539-1450 (Print) 1539-1450 (Linking)

Grewe, J.M., Cervenka, J., Shapiro, B.L. & Witkop, C.J., Jr. (1968). Prevalence o f malocclusion in Chippewa Indian children. *Journal of dental research,* Vol. 47, No. 2, (Mar-Apr 1968), pp. 302-305, 0022-0345 (Print) 0022-0345 (Linking)

Grumbach, M.M. (2000). Estrogen, bone, growth and sex: a sea change in conventional wisdom. *J Pediatr Endocrinol Metab,* Vol. 13 Suppl 6, No. 2000), pp. 1439-1455, 0334-018X (Print)

Gu, Y. & McNamara, J.A. (2007). Mandibular growth changes and cervical vertebral maturation. a cephalometric implant study. *The Angle orthodontist,* Vol. 77, No. 6, (Nov 2007), pp. 947-953, 0003-3219 (Print)

Guo, Y., Xiong, D.H., Yang, T.L., Guo, Y.F., Recker, R.R. & Deng, H.W. (2006). Polymorphisms of estrogen-biosynthesis genes CYP17 and CYP19 may influence age at menarche: a genetic association study in Caucasian females. *Human molecular genetics,* Vol. 15, No. 16, (Aug 15 2006), pp. 2401-2408, 0964-6906 (Print)

Harris, E.F. & Smith, R.J. (1980). A study of occlusion and arch widths in families. *American journal of orthodontics,* Vol. 78, No. 2, (Aug 1980), pp. 155-163, 0002-9416 (Print)

Harris, E.F. & Johnson, M.G. (1991). Heritability of craniometric and occlusal variables: a longitudinal sib analysis. *American journal of orthodontics and dentofacial orthopedics : official publication of the American Association of Orthodontists, its constituent societies, and the American Board of Orthodontics,* Vol. 99, No. 3, (Mar 1991), pp. 258-268, 0889-5406 (Print)

Harris, E.F. & Potter, R.H. (1997). Sources of bias in heritability studies. *American journal of orthodontics and dentofacial orthopedics : official publication of the American Association of Orthodontists, its constituent societies, and the American Board of Orthodontics,* Vol. 112, No. 3, (Sep 1997), pp. 17A-21A, 0889-5406 (Print)

Harris, E.F. (2008). Interpreting Heritability Estimates in the Orthodontic Literature. *Semin Orthod,* Vol. 14, No. 2008), pp. 125-134,

Harris, J.E., Kowalski, C.J. & Watnick, S.S. (1973). Genetic factors in the shape of the craniofacial complex. *The Angle orthodontist,* Vol. 43, No. 1, (Jan 1973), pp. 107-111, 0003-3219 (Print)

Harris, J.E., Kowalski, C.J. & Walker, S.J. (1975). Intrafamilial dentofacial associations for Class II, Division 1 probands. *American journal of orthodontics*, Vol. 67, No. 5, (May 1975), pp. 563-570, 0002-9416 (Print)

Harris, J.E. & Kowalski, C.J. (1976). All in the family: use of familial information in orthodontic diagnosis, case assessment, and treatment planning. *American journal of orthodontics*, Vol. 69, No. 5, (May 1976), pp. 493-510, 0002-9416 (Print)

Hartsfield, J.K., Jr. (2008). Personalized Orthodontics, The Future of Genetics in Practice. *Semin Orthod*, Vol. 14, No. 2008), pp. 166-171,

Hartsfield, J.K., Jr., Zhou, J. & Chen, S. (2010).In: *Surgical Enhancement of Orthodontic Treatment, Craniofacial Growth Series, Department of Orthodontics and Pediatric Dentistry and Center for Human Growth and Development*, J.A. McNamara & S.D. Kapila, pp. 267-281, The University of Michigan,Ann Arbor

Hartsfield, J.K., Jr. (2011).5, In: *Orthodontics : current principles and techniques*, L.W. Graber, R.L. Vanarsdall & K.W.L. Vig, pp. 139-156, Elsevier Mosby,0323066410 St Louis

Hartsfield, J.K., Jr. & Bixler, D. (2011).6, In: *McDonald's and Avery's dentistry for the child and adolescent*, J.A. Dean, D.R. Avery & R.E. McDonald, pp. 64-84, Mosby/Elsevier,9780323057240, St. Louis, Mo.

Hartsfield Jr., J.K., Zhou, J. & Chen, S. (2010). Genetic Variation in the CYP19A1/Aromatase Gene and Facial Growth. *Journal of dental research*, Vol. 89, No. Special Issue A, 2010), pp. Abstract 63, (www.dentalresearch.org).

Hashim, H.A. & Sarhan, O.A. (1993). Dento-skeletal components of class III malocclusions for children with normal and protruded mandibles. *The Journal of clinical pediatric dentistry*, Vol. 18, No. 1, (Fall 1993), pp. 12-16, 1053-4628 (Print) 1053-4628 (Linking)

Hashim, H.A. & Al-Ghamdi, S. (2005). Tooth width and arch dimensions in normal and malocclusion samples: an odontometric study. *J Contemp Dent Pract*, Vol. 6, No. 2, (May 15 2005), pp. 36-51, 1526-3711 (Electronic) 1526-3711 (Linking)

Hauspie, R.C., Susanne, C. & Defrise-Gussenhoven, E. (1985). Testing for the presence of genetic variance in factors of face measurements of Belgian twins. *Annals of human biology*, Vol. 12, No. 5, (Sep-Oct 1985), pp. 429-440, 0301-4460 (Print)

He, S., Hartsfield, J., Guo, Y., Cao, Y., Wang, S. & Chen, S. (2011). *Association between CYP19A1 SNPs and haplotypes and pubertal sagittal jaw growth*, Submitted to the Journal of Dental Research.

Helm, S. (1968). Malocclusion in Danish children with adolescent dentition: an epidemiologic study. *American journal of orthodontics*, Vol. 54, No. 5, (May 1968), pp. 352-366, 0002-9416 (Print) 0002-9416 (Linking)

Hennekam, R.C.M., Allanson, J.E., Krantz, I.D. & Gorlin, R.J. (2010). *Gorlin's syndromes of the head and neck* (edition), Oxford University Press, 9780195307900 (alk. paper), Oxford; New York

Honjo, H., Tamura, T., Matsumoto, Y., Kawata, M., Ogino, Y., Tanaka, K., Yamamoto, T., Ueda, S. & Okada, H. (1992). Estrogen as a growth factor to central nervous cells. Estrogen treatment promotes development of acetylcholinesterase-positive basal forebrain neurons transplanted in the anterior eye chamber. *J Steroid Biochem Mol Biol*, Vol. 41, No. 3-8, (Mar 1992), pp. 633-635, 0960-0760 (Print)

Horowitz, H.S. (1970). A study of occlusal relations in 10 to 12 year old Caucasian and Negro children--summary report. *International dental journal,* Vol. 20, No. 4, (Dec 1970), pp. 593-605, 0020-6539 (Print) 0020-6539 (Linking)

Horowitz, S.L., Osborne, R.H. & DeGeorge, F.V. (1960). A Cephalometric Study Of Craniofacial Variation In Adult Twins. *The Angle orthodontist,* Vol. 30, No. 1, 1960), pp. 1-5,

Hunter, W.S., Balbach, D.R. & Lamphiear, D.E. (1970). The heritability of attained growth in the human face. *American journal of orthodontics,* Vol. 58, No. 2, (Aug 1970), pp. 128-134, 0002-9416 (Print) 0002-9416 (Linking)

Hunter, W.S. (1990). *Heredity in the craniofacial complex.* (edition), Saunders, Philadelphia

Hunter, W.S., Baumrind, S., Popovich, F. & Jorgensen, G. (2007). Forecasting the timing of peak mandibular growth in males by using skeletal age. *American journal of orthodontics and dentofacial orthopedics : official publication of the American Association of Orthodontists, its constituent societies, and the American Board of Orthodontics,* Vol. 131, No. 3, (Mar 2007), pp. 327-333, 1097-6752 (Electronic)

Ingervall, B. (1974). Prevalence of dental and occlusal anomalies in Swedish conscripts. *Acta odontologica Scandinavica,* Vol. 32, No. 2, 1974), pp. 83-92, 0001-6357 (Print) 0001-6357 (Linking)

Ishii, N., Deguchi, T. & Hunt, N.P. (2002). Craniofacial differences between Japanese and British Caucasian females with a skeletal Class III malocclusion. *European journal of orthodontics,* Vol. 24, No. 5, (Oct 2002), pp. 493-499, 0141-5387 (Print) 0141-5387 (Linking)

Jang, J.Y., Park, E.K., Ryoo, H.M., Shin, H.I., Kim, T.H., Jang, J.S., Park, H.S., Choi, J.Y. & Kwon, T.G. (2010). Polymorphisms in the Matrilin-1 gene and risk of mandibular prognathism in Koreans. *Journal of dental research,* Vol. 89, No. 11, (Nov 2010), pp. 1203-1207, 1544-0591 (Electronic) 0022-0345 (Linking)

Johannsdottir, B., Thorarinsson, F., Thordarson, A. & Magnusson, T.E. (2005). Heritability of craniofacial characteristics between parents and offspring estimated from lateral cephalograms. *American journal of orthodontics and dentofacial orthopedics : official publication of the American Association of Orthodontists, its constituent societies, and the American Board of Orthodontics,* Vol. 127, No. 2, (Feb 2005), pp. 200-207; quiz 260-201, 0889-5406 (Print) 0889-5406 (Linking)

Kang, E.H., Yamaguchi, T., Tajima, A., Nakajima, T., Tomoyasu, Y., Watanabe, M., Yamaguchi, M., Park, S.B., Maki, K. & Inoue, I. (2009). Association of the growth hormone receptor gene polymorphisms with mandibular height in a Korean population. *Archives of oral biology,* Vol. 54, No. 6, (Jun 2009), pp. 556-562, 1879-1506 (Electronic) 0003-9969 (Linking)

Kawala, B., Antoszewska, J. & Necka, A. (2007). Genetics or environment? A twin-method study of malocclusions. *World journal of orthodontics,* Vol. 8, No. 4, (Winter 2007), pp. 405-410, 1530-5678 (Print) 1530-5678 (Linking)

King, L., Harris, E.F. & Tolley, E.A. (1993). Heritability of cephalometric and occlusal variables as assessed from siblings with overt malocclusions. *American journal of orthodontics and dentofacial orthopedics : official publication of the American Association of*

Orthodontists, its constituent societies, and the American Board of Orthodontics, Vol. 104, No. 2, (Aug 1993), pp. 121-131, 0889-5406 (Print)

Klingenberg, C.P., Leamy, L.J. & Cheverud, J.M. (2004). Integration and modularity of quantitative trait locus effects on geometric shape in the mouse mandible. *Genetics*, Vol. 166, No. 4, (Apr 2004), pp. 1909-1921, 0016-6731 (Print) 0016-6731 (Linking)

Kraus, B.S., Wise, W.J. & Frei, R.H. (1959). Heredity and the craniofacial complex. *American journal of orthodontics*, Vol. 45, No. 1959), pp. 172,

Kraus, P. & Lufkin, T. (2006). Dlx homeobox gene control of mammalian limb and craniofacial development. *American journal of medical genetics. Part A*, Vol. 140, No. 13, (Jul 1 2006), pp. 1366-1374, 1552-4825 (Print) 1552-4825 (Linking)

Krauss, B., Wise, W. & Frei, R. (1959). Heredity and the craniofacial complex. *American journal of orthodontics*, Vol. 45, No. 1959), pp. 172-217,

Laine, T. & Hausen, H. (1983). Occlusal anomalies in Finnish students related to age, sex, absent permanent teeth and orthodontic treatment. *European journal of orthodontics*, Vol. 5, No. 2, (May 1983), pp. 125-131, 0141-5387 (Print) 0141-5387 (Linking)

Lambert, M.-P. & Herceg, Z. (2011). *Mechanisms of Epigenetic Gene Silencing*, Epigenetic Aspects of Chronic Diseases. H.I. Roach, F. Bronner & R.O.C. Oreffo. Springer, London. 41-53

Lavelle, C.L. (1983). Study of mandibular shape in the mouse. *Acta Anat (Basel)*, Vol. 117, No. 4, 1983), pp. 314-320, 0001-5180 (Print)

Li, Q., Zhang, F., Li, X. & Chen, F. (2010). Genome scan for locus involved in mandibular prognathism in pedigrees from China. *PLoS One*, Vol. 5, No. 9, 2010), pp. 1932-6203 (Electronic) 1932-6203 (Linking)

Li, Q., Li, X., Zhang, F. & Chen, F. (2011). The identification of a novel locus for mandibular prognathism in the Han Chinese population. *Journal of dental research*, Vol. 90, No. 1, (Jan 2011), pp. 53-57, 1544-0591 (Electronic) 0022-0345 (Linking)

Litton, S.F., Ackermann, L.V., Isaacson, R.J. & Shapiro, B.L. (1970). A genetic study of Class 3 malocclusion. *American journal of orthodontics*, Vol. 58, No. 6, (Dec 1970), pp. 565-577, 0002-9416 (Print) 0002-9416 (Linking)

Lobb, W.K. (1987). Craniofacial morphology and occlusal variation in monozygous and dizygous twins. *The Angle orthodontist*, Vol. 57, No. 3, (Jul 1987), pp. 219-233, 0003-3219 (Print) 0003-3219 (Linking)

Luffingham, J.K. & Campbell, H.M. (1974). The need for orthodontic treatment. A pilot survey of 14 year old school children in Paisley, Scotland. *Transactions. European Orthodontic Society*, Vol. No. 1974), pp. 259-267,

Lundstrom, A. & McWilliam, J.S. (1987). A comparison of vertical and horizontal cephalometric variables with regard to heritability. *European journal of orthodontics*, Vol. 9, No. 2, (May 1987), pp. 104-108, 0141-5387 (Print)

Mackay, F., Jones, J.A., Thompson, R. & Simpson, W. (1992). Craniofacial form in class III cases. *British journal of orthodontics*, Vol. 19, No. 1, (Feb 1992), pp. 15-20, 0301-228X (Print) 0301-228X (Linking)

Malinowski, A. (1983). Changes in dimensions and proportions of the human mandible during fetal period. *Collegium antropologicum*, Vol. 7, No. 1983), pp. 65-70,

Manfredi, C., Martina, R., Grossi, G.B. & Giuliani, M. (1997). Heritability of 39 orthodontic cephalometric parameters on MZ, DZ twins and MN-paired singletons. *American journal of orthodontics and dentofacial orthopedics : official publication of the American Association of Orthodontists, its constituent societies, and the American Board of Orthodontics,* Vol. 111, No. 1, (Jan 1997), pp. 44-51, 0889-5406 (Print) 0889-5406 (Linking)

Maor, G., Segev, Y. & Phillip, M. (1999). Testosterone stimulates insulin-like growth factor-I and insulin-like growth factor-I-receptor gene expression in the mandibular condyle--a model of endochondral ossification. *Endocrinology,* Vol. 140, No. 4, (Apr 1999), pp. 1901-1910, 0013-7227 (Print) 0013-7227 (Linking)

Markovic, M.D. (1992). At the crossroads of oral facial genetics. *European journal of orthodontics,* Vol. 14, No. 6, (Dec 1992), pp. 469-481, 0141-5387 (Print) 0141-5387 (Linking)

Martins Mda, G. & Lima, K.C. (2009). Prevalence of malocclusions in 10- to 12-year-old schoolchildren in Ceara, Brazil. *Oral health & preventive dentistry,* Vol. 7, No. 3, 2009), pp. 217-223, 1602-1622 (Print) 1602-1622 (Linking)

Martone, V.D., Enlow, D.H., Hans, M.G., Broadbent, B.H., Jr. & Oyen, O. (1992). Class I and Class III malocclusion sub-groupings related to headform type. *The Angle orthodontist,* Vol. 62, No. 1, (Spring 1992), pp. 35-42; discussion 43-34, 0003-3219 (Print) 0003-3219 (Linking)

Massler, M. & Frankel, J.M. (1951). Prevalence of malocclusion in children aged 14 to 18 years. *American journal of orthodontics,* Vol. 37, No. 10, (Oct 1951), pp. 751-768, 0002-9416 (Print) 0002-9416 (Linking)

Mills, L.F. (1966). Epidemiologic studies of occlusion. IV. The prevalence of malocclusion in a population of 1,455 school children. *Journal of dental research,* Vol. 45, No. 2, (Mar-Apr 1966), pp. 332-336, 0022-0345

Morford, L.A., Coles, T.J., Fardo, D.W., Wall, M.D., Morrison, M.W., Kula, K.S. & Hartsfield, J.K., Jr. (2010a). Assocaiton analysis of Class II division 2 (CII/D2) with RUNX2 and RUNX3 Journal of dental research. 89 (Special Iss B) abstract #1948:

Morford, L.A., Wall, M.D., Morrison, M.W., Kula, K.S. & Hartsfield, J.K., Jr. (2010b). *Association Analysis of Class-II Division-2 (CII/D2) with PAX9 and MSX1,* Journal of dental research. 89 (Special Iss A) abstract #633:

Morrison, M.W. (2008). *Relative Risk of Class II division 2 Malocclusion in First-Degree Relatives of Probands with Class II division 2 Malocclusion,* Department of Orthodontics and Oral Facial Genetics. Indiana University School of Dentistry, Master of Science in Dentistry degree:

Moss, M.L. (1997a). The functional matrix hypothesis revisited. 4. The epigenetic antithesis and the resolving synthesis. *American journal of orthodontics and dentofacial orthopedics : official publication of the American Association of Orthodontists, its constituent societies, and the American Board of Orthodontics,* Vol. 112, No. 4, 1997a), pp. 410-417.,

Moss, M.L. (1997b). The functional matrix hypothesis revisited. 3. The genomic thesis. *American journal of orthodontics and dentofacial orthopedics : official publication of the*

American Association of Orthodontists, its constituent societies, and the American Board of Orthodontics, Vol. 112, No. 3, 1997b), pp. 338-342.,

Mossey, P.A. (1999a). The heritability of malocclusion: Part 1--Genetics, principles and terminology. *British journal of orthodontics,* Vol. 26, No. 2, (Jun 1999a), pp. 103-113, 0301-228X (Print)

Mossey, P.A. (1999b). The heritability of malocclusion: part 2. The influence of genetics in malocclusion. *British journal of orthodontics,* Vol. 26, No. 3, (Sep 1999b), pp. 195-203, 0301-228X (Print) 0301-228X (Linking)

Nakasima, A., Ichinose, M., Nakata, S. & Takahama, Y. (1982). Hereditary factors in the craniofacial morphology of Angle's Class II and Class III malocclusions. *American journal of orthodontics,* Vol. 82, No. 2, (Aug 1982), pp. 150-156, 0002-9416 (Print) 0002-9416 (Linking)

Nakata, N., Yu, P.I., Davis, B. & Nance, W.E. (1973). The use of genetic data in the prediction of craniofacial dimensions. *American journal of orthodontics,* Vol. 63, No. 5, (May 1973), pp. 471-480, 0002-9416 (Print) 0002-9416 (Linking)

Nikolova, M. (1996). Similarities in anthropometrical traits of children and their parents in a Bulgarian population. *Annals of human genetics,* Vol. 60, No. Pt 6, (Nov 1996), pp. 517-525, 0003-4800 (Print) 0003-4800 (Linking)

Niswander, J.D. (1975). Genetics of common dental disorders. *Dent Clin North Am,* Vol. 19, No. 1, (Jan 1975), pp. 197-206, 0011-8532 (Print)

Peck, S., Peck, L. & Kataja, M. (1998). Class II Division 2 malocclusion: a heritable pattern of small teeth in well-developed jaws. *The Angle orthodontist,* Vol. 68, No. 1, (Feb 1998), pp. 9-20, 0003-3219

Poosti, M. & Jalali, T. (2007). Tooth size and arch dimension in uncrowded versus crowded Class I malocclusions. *J Contemp Dent Pract,* Vol. 8, No. 3, 2007), pp. 45-52, 1526-3711 (Electronic) 1526-3711 (Linking)

Proffit, W.R. (1986). On the aetiology of malocclusion. The Northcroft lecture, 1985 presented to the British Society for the Study of Orthodontics, Oxford, April 18, 1985. *British journal of orthodontics,* Vol. 13, No. 1, (Jan 1986), pp. 1-11, 0301-228X (Print)

Ruf, S. & Pancherz, H. (1999). Class II Division 2 malocclusion: genetics or environment? A case report of monozygotic twins. *The Angle orthodontist,* Vol. 69, No. 4, (Aug 1999), pp. 321-324, 0003-3219

Saleh, F.K. (1999). Prevalence of malocclusion in a sample of Lebanese schoolchildren: an epidemiological study. *Eastern Mediterranean health journal = La revue de sante de la Mediterranee orientale = al-Majallah al-sihhiyah li-sharq al-mutawassit,* Vol. 5, No. 2, (Mar 1999), pp. 337-343, 1020-3397 (Print) 1020-3397 (Linking)

Sasaki, Y., Satoh, K., Hayasaki, H., Fukumoto, S., Fujiwara, T. & Nonaka, K. (2009). The P561T polymorphism of the growth hormone receptor gene has an inhibitory effect on mandibular growth in young children. *European journal of orthodontics,* Vol. 31, No. 5, (Oct 2009), pp. 536-541, 1460-2210 (Electronic) 0141-5387 (Linking)

Saunders, S.R., Popovich, F. & Thompson, G.W. (1980). A family study of craniofacial dimensions in the Burlington Growth Centre sample. *American journal of*

orthodontics, Vol. 78, No. 4, (Oct 1980), pp. 394-403, 0002-9416 (Print) 0002-9416
(Linking)

Schaefer, K., Fink, B., Mitteroecker, P., Neave, N. & Bookstein, F.L. (2005). Visualizing facial
shape regression upon 2nd to 4th digit ratio and testosterone. Collegium
antropologicum, Vol. 29, No. 2, (Dec 2005), pp. 415-419, 0350-6134 (Print) 0350-6134
(Linking)

Schaefer, K., Fink, B., Grammer, K., Mitteroecker, P., Gunz, P. & Bookstein, F.L. (2006).
Female appearance: facial and bodily attractiveness as shape. Psych Sci, Vol. 48, No.
2006), pp. 187-204,

Schwartz, D.A. (2010). Epigenetics and environmental lung disease. Proceedings of the
American Thoracic Society, Vol. 7, No. 2, (May 2010), pp. 123-125, 1943-5665
(Electronic) 1546-3222 (Linking)

Singh, G.D. (1999). Morphologic determinants in the etiology of class III malocclusions: a
review. Clinical anatomy, Vol. 12, No. 5, 1999), pp. 382-405, 0897-3806 (Print) 0897-
3806 (Linking)

Solow, B. & Helm, S. (1968). A method for tabulation and statistical evaluation of
epidemiological malocclusion data. Acta odontologica Scandinavica, Vol. 26, No. 1,
(May 1968), pp. 63-88, 0001-6357 (Print) 0001-6357 (Linking)

Stiles, K. & Luke, J. (1953). The inheritance of malocclusion due to mandibular prognathism.
J of Hereditary, Vol. 44, No. 1953), pp. 241-245,

Strohmayer, W. (1937). Die Vereburg des Hapsburger Familientypus. Nova Acta Leopoldina,
Vol. 5, No. 1937), pp. 219-296,

Susanne, C. & Sharma, P.D. (1978). Multivariate analysis of head measurements in Punjabi
families. Annals of human biology, Vol. 5, No. 2, (Mar 1978), pp. 179-183, 0301-4460
(Print)

Suzuki, S. (1961). Studies on the so-called reverse occlusion. The Journal of Nihon University
School of Dentistry, Vol. 3, No. 1961), pp. 51-58,

Tassopoulou-Fishell, M., Deeley, K., Harvey, E., Sciote, J. & Viera, A. (2011). MYO1H
contributes to Class III malocclusion. Journal of dental research, Vol. 90 (Special Iss A)
abstract #248, No. 2011), pp.

Thesleff, I. (2006). The genetic basis of tooth development and dental defects. American
journal of medical genetics. Part A, Vol. 140, No. 23, (Dec 1 2006), pp. 2530-2535, 1552-
4825 (Print) 1552-4825 (Linking)

Thilander, B., Pena, L., Infante, C., Parada, S.S. & de Mayorga, C. (2001). Prevalence of
malocclusion and orthodontic treatment need in children and adolescents in
Bogota, Colombia. An epidemiological study related to different stages of dental
development. European journal of orthodontics, Vol. 23, No. 2, (Apr 2001), pp. 153-
167, 0141-5387 (Print) 0141-5387 (Linking)

Thompson, E.M. & Winter, R.M. (1988). Another family with the 'Habsburg jaw'. Journal of
medical genetics, Vol. 25, No. 12, (Dec 1988), pp. 838-842, 0022-2593 (Print) 0022-2593
(Linking)

Ting, T.Y., Wong, R.W. & Rabie, A.B. (2011). Analysis of genetic polymorphisms in skeletal
Class I crowding. American journal of orthodontics and dentofacial orthopedics : official
publication of the American Association of Orthodontists, its constituent societies, and the

American Board of Orthodontics, Vol. 140, No. 1, (Jul 2011), pp. e9-15, 1097-6752 (Electronic) 0889-5406 (Linking)

Tipton, R.T. & Rinchuse, D.J. (1991). The relationship between static occlusion and functional occlusion in a dental school population. *The Angle orthodontist,* Vol. 61, No. 1, (Spring 1991), pp. 57-66, 0003-3219 (Print) 0003-3219 (Linking)

Tomoyasu, Y., Yamaguchi, T., Tajima, A., Nakajima, T., Inoue, I. & Maki, K. (2009). Further evidence for an association between mandibular height and the growth hormone receptor gene in a Japanese population. *American journal of orthodontics and dentofacial orthopedics : official publication of the American Association of Orthodontists, its constituent societies, and the American Board of Orthodontics,* Vol. 136, No. 4, (Oct 2009), pp. 536-541, 1097-6752 (Electronic) 0889-5406 (Linking)

Townsend, G., Richards, L. & Hughes, T. (2003). Molar intercuspal dimensions: genetic input to phenotypic variation. *Journal of dental research,* Vol. 82, No. 5, (May 2003), pp. 350-355, 0022-0345 (Print)

Turchetta, B.J., Fishman, L.S. & Subtelny, J.D. (2007). Facial growth prediction: a comparison of methodologies. *American journal of orthodontics and dentofacial orthopedics : official publication of the American Association of Orthodontists, its constituent societies, and the American Board of Orthodontics,* Vol. 132, No. 4, (Oct 2007), pp. 439-449, 1097-6752 (Electronic)

Verdonck, A., De Ridder, L., Verbeke, G., Bourguignon, J.P., Carels, C., Kuhn, E.R., Darras, V. & de Zegher, F. (1998). Comparative effects of neonatal and prepubertal castration on craniofacial growth in rats. *Archives of oral biology,* Vol. 43, No. 11, (Nov 1998), pp. 861-871, 0003-9969 (Print) 0003-9969 (Linking)

Verdonck, A., Gaethofs, M., Carels, C. & de Zegher, F. (1999). Effect of low-dose testosterone treatment on craniofacial growth in boys with delayed puberty. *European journal of orthodontics,* Vol. 21, No. 2, (Apr 1999), pp. 137-143, 0141-5387 (Print) 0141-5387 (Linking)

Verma, D., Peltomaki, T. & Jager, A. (2009). Reliability of growth prediction with hand-wrist radiographs. *European journal of orthodontics,* Vol. 31, No. 4, (Aug 2009), pp. 438-442, 1460-2210 (Electronic)

Watnick, S.S. (1972). Inheritance of craniofacial morphology. *The Angle orthodontist,* Vol. 42, No. 4, (Oct 1972), pp. 339-351, 0003-3219 (Print) 0003-3219 (Linking)

Wolff, G., Wienker, T.F. & Sander, H. (1993). On the genetics of mandibular prognathism: analysis of large European noble families. *Journal of medical genetics,* Vol. 30, No. 2, (Feb 1993), pp. 112-116, 0022-2593 (Print) 0022-2593 (Linking)

Xue, F., Wong, R.W. & Rabie, A.B. (2010). Genes, genetics, and Class III malocclusion. *Orthodontics & craniofacial research,* Vol. 13, No. 2, (May 2010), pp. 69-74, 1601-6343 (Electronic) 1601-6335 (Linking)

Yamaguchi, T., Maki, K. & Shibasaki, Y. (2001). Growth hormone receptor gene variant and mandibular height in the normal Japanese population. *American journal of orthodontics and dentofacial orthopedics : official publication of the American Association of Orthodontists, its constituent societies, and the American Board of Orthodontics,* Vol. 119, No. 6, (Jun 2001), pp. 650-653, 0889-5406 (Print)

Yamaguchi, T., Park, S.B., Narita, A., Maki, K. & Inoue, I. (2005). Genome-wide linkage
        analysis of mandibular prognathism in Korean and Japanese patients. *Journal of
        dental research,* Vol. 84, No. 3, (Mar 2005), pp. 255-259, 0022-0345 (Print) 0022-0345
        (Linking)
Zammit, M.P., Hans, M.G., Broadbent, B.H., Johnsen, D.C., Latimer, B.M. & Nelson, S.
        (1995). Malocclusion in Labrador Inuit youth: a psychosocial, dental and
        cephalometric evaluation. *Arctic medical research,* Vol. 54, No. 1, (Jan 1995), pp. 32-
        44, 0782-226X (Print) 0782-226X (Linking)

8

Three-Dimensional Imaging and Software Advances in Orthodontics

Ahmed Ghoneima[1,2], Eman Allam[1], Katherine Kula[1] and L. Jack Windsor[1]
[1]Indiana University School of Dentistry, Indianapolis,
[2]Faculty of Dental Medicine, Al-Azhar University, Cairo
[1]USA
[2]Egypt

1. Introduction

The technological advances and innovations of imaging systems for orthodontic practice require a continuous update of their applications and assessments of their strength and weakness, as well as guidelines for utilization. Orthodontists are challenged by the increasing number and complexity of these systems and softwares. Accurate diagnostic imaging is an essential requirement for the optimal diagnosis and treatment planning of orthodontic patients. In addition, it is a critical tool that allows the clinician to monitor and document the treatment progress and outcome. The purpose of this chapter is to update orthodontists about the current options and applications of the latest imaging techniques in orthodontic practice and to review the existing software advances.

2. Cone beam technology in orthodontics

The cone-beam computed tomography (CBCT) scanners were introduced in the late 1990s. Shortly after, the US Food and Drug Administration (FDA) approved the first CBCT unit in 2001. Since then, there has been an enormous interest in this new technology for its clinical and research applications. The CBCT is an imaging acquisition technique that utilizes a volumetric scanning machine. This technology is based on a cone-shaped X-ray beam directed at a flat two-dimensional (2D) detector. As both rotate around the patient's head, a series of 2D images are generated. The software then reconstructs the images into three-dimensional (3D) data set using a specialized algorithm (De Vos et al., 2009; Molen, 2011).

Currently, there are more than 43 CBCT systems from 20 different companies available commercially. The most commonly used of these CBCT imaging aquistion systems are the 3D Accuitomo (J. Morita, Kyoto, Japan), CB MercuRay (Hitachi Medical Corporation, Osaka, Japan), iCAT (Imaging Sciences International, Hatfield, PA), Galileos (Sirona Dental Systems LLC, Charlotte, NC), New-Tom 3G (QR srl, Verona, Italy), Scanora 3D (SOREDEX, Milwaukee, WI), and Kodak 9500 (Kodak Dental Systems, Rochester, NY). There are big variations in the quality and characteristics of the images or the reconstructed volumes and the radiation doses between most of these CBCT systems. Machines with reduced radiation doses and less powerful tubes are often associated with poor image quality, low contrast resolution and increased noise. The exposure parameters, the source-detector distance, the field of view (FOV), the data reconstruction algorithm, and the software used are among the major factors responsible for those variations. The currently available CBCT units utilize radiation doses ranging from 87 to 206 µSv for a full craniofacial scan. These radiation doses are slightly higher than the conventional radiographic techniques such as the lateral cephalograms or the panoramic radiographs and markedly lower than that of multi-slice CT. The scan time varies between 10 to 75 seconds, depending on the FOV and the CBCT unit used (Molen, 2011; Kapila et al., 2011).

Craniofacial imaging is a crucial component of an orthodontic patient's record. The gold standard for orthodontic records is the attempt to achieve an accurate replication of the real anatomical structures or the "anatomic truth". Although the use of the traditional imaging views in orthodontics has been adequate, the achievement of the ideal imaging goal of replicating the anatomic truth has been limited by the available technology such as the 2D frontal and lateral cephalograms, panoramic radiographs, and intraoral/extraoral photographs. Recently, more emphasis has been placed on the CBCT technology, the 3D images, and virtual models. The main advantage for the use of CBCT is that the clinician can get more accurate data from one scan than from the many 2D radiographs traditionally used with less radiation exposure (Mah & Hatcher, 2005) (Figure 1).

The 3D CBCT data can greatly expand the orthodontist's diagnostic capabilities. It offers a comprehensive evaluation of the dentition and is very useful for identifying abnormalities such as missing teeth, supernumerary teeth, eruption disturbances, teeth malpositions, and/or root irregularities that could delay or prevent tooth movement. CBCT can be considered the technique of choice for examining and localizing impacted teeth. The exact position of impacted tooth and its relations to the adjacent roots or important anatomical structures such as the maxillary sinus or the mandibular canal when planning surgical exposure and subsequently orthodontic management can be precisely assessed by 3D CBCT (Mah et al., 2011) (Figures 2 and 3).

Using CBCT scans, alveolar bone can be assessed from all aspects not only on the mesial and distal surfaces of the tooth. This allows for the assessment of the width of available bone for buccolingual movement of teeth during orthodontic management especially in cases requiring arch expansion or labial movement of incisors. Fenestrations, dehiscence, and/or external apical root resorption can be precisely visualized on the 3D images. Evaluation of alveolar bone volume, which is especially important in periodontally compromised adult orthodontic patients, is one of the beneficial uses of CBCT in orthodontics. The width of alveolar ridges for placement of implants is another variable that can be investigated (Halazonetis, 2005; Valiathan et al., 2008).

Preoperative implant site assessment is probably one of the most useful applications of CBCT in orthodontics. In the orthodontic field, osseo-integrated implants are either used for anchorage or as a prosthetic replacement of missing teeth. The accurate determination of root angulations and the available space are essential for successful placement of the implant. CBCT can be used to accurately assess the space availability and root angulation, as well as the 3D quantification of the alveolar bone at the implant site (Mah & Hatcher, 2005) (Figure 4).

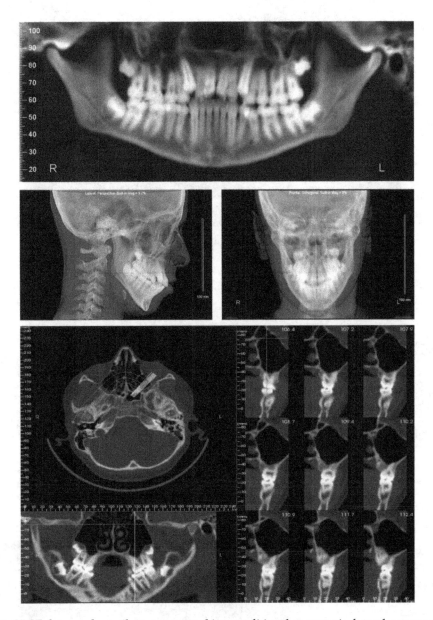

Fig. 1. CBCT data can be easily reconstructed into traditional panoramic, lateral, or postero-anterior cephalometric images, as well as cross section views. In this way, the clinician can get more information from the scan than from multiple 2D radiographs with less radiation exposure. Images created by the Dolphin and InVivoDental softwares from a single CBCT scan.

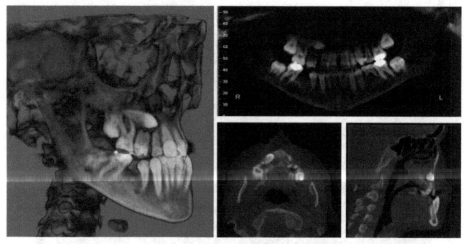

Fig. 2. A 15 years old female with impacted canine that was initially diagnosed on the panoramic radiograph, but could not be precisely located in relationship to the present teeth. Using the axial and sagittal sections of the CBCT data, the labial location could be confirmed. In addition, the 3D volume allowed for viewing the impacted canine from any angle.

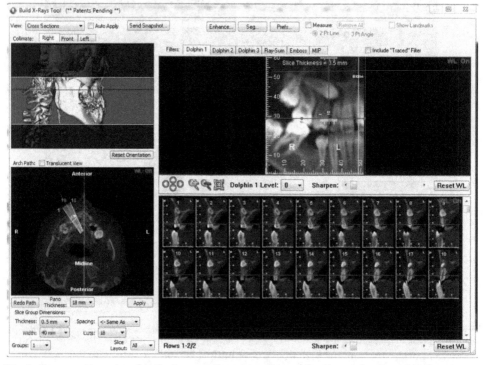

Fig. 3. Cross section view for the impacted canine allowed for the evaluation of its location and relationship to other structures slice by slice in 1 view (slice thickness 0.5 mm).

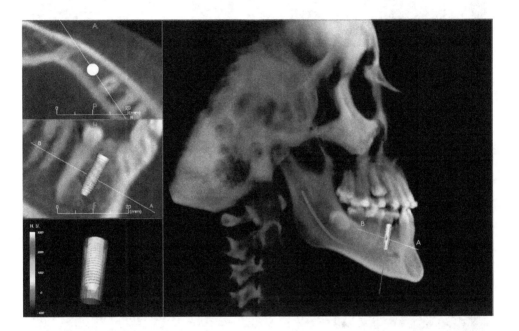

Fig. 4. Axial and sagittal sections showing the buccal and lingual bone thickness, as well as the relationship between the implant and the inferior alveolar nerve (labeled in red color). The 3D view is important in the evaluation of space availability.

Orthodontic patients with temporomandibular joint (TMJ) disorders are common. When these disorders occur during development, they may alter the facial growth pattern and may also affect the growth of the ipsilateral part of the mandible with compensations in the maxilla, tooth position, occlusion, and cranial base. CBCT allows the clinicians to assess and quantify these changes associated with TMJ disorders more accurately than the 2D images as these changes occur in the vertical, horizontal, and transverse directions. CBCT is especially indicated when more information about the morphology and internal structure of the osseous components of the TMJ is required. Studies have shown that CBCT images provide higher reliability and accuracy than CT and panoramic radiographs in the detection of condylar cortical erosion. CBCT images also allow for the visualization of the TMJs from different views and efficient evaluation of its relationship to the dentition and occlusion (Huang, et al., 2005; Hilgers et al., 2005; Honey et al., 2007) (Figure 5).

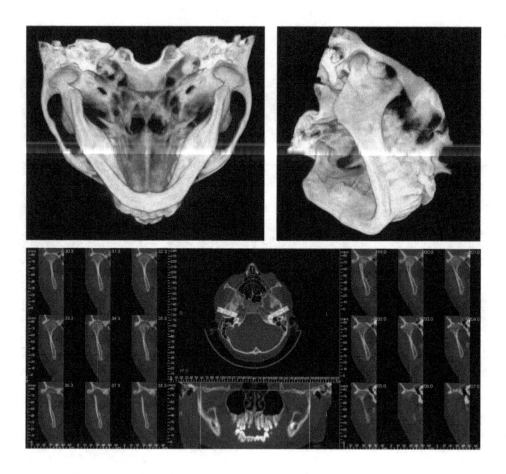

Fig. 5. 3D CBCT volume allows for better visualization and provides more details about the morphology and position of the TMJ and the condyles from different views. In addition, the TMJ cross-section view permits complete and thorough examination of the joint through a group of cross section slices.

Digital study models have been introduced as the digital alternative to the traditional stone cast record. A gradual transition from the plaster models decade to the digital models is expected to occur in the near future. The rapid growth and acceptance of these digital models among the orthodontists has been driven by many factors. They are easier and faster to obtain, to store, transfer, and retrieve. Patients benefit from shorter appointment time when impressions are not needed, and the clinicians benefit from the superior diagnosis and treatment simulation provided by better presentation of the dentition and manipulation of the images (Enciso et al., 2003).

The digital models allow the clinician to obtain additional diagnostic information that are not available with the use of the plaster models such as root shape, position, and angulations. The relationship of the roots to anatomic structures such as the mandibular nerve, as well as quantitative bone density information, can also be evaluated. Crown to root ratios can be estimated and other different dental measurements can be performed easily. Several studies have proved that the digital models created from CBCT scans or obtained from laser scanning of a dental impression or study model are as accurate and as reliable as plasters models (Dalstra & Melsen, 2009; Hernandez-Soler et al., 2011). Perhaps a major advantage of the digital models is the virtual setup capability with complete 3D anatomy by including the roots and the alveolar bone. The virtual setup provides superior case presentation, treatment simulation, aesthetic predictions, and results visualization. It also allows for including the torque and labiolingual inclination calculations in the dental setup (Hernandez-Soler et al., 2011) (Figures 6 and 7).

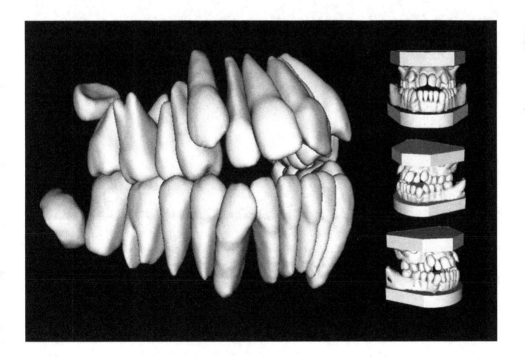

Fig. 6. Computer-generated models reconstructed from the digital imaging and communications in medicine (DICOM) data using the InVivoDental software showing not only the crowns of the teeth but also the roots.

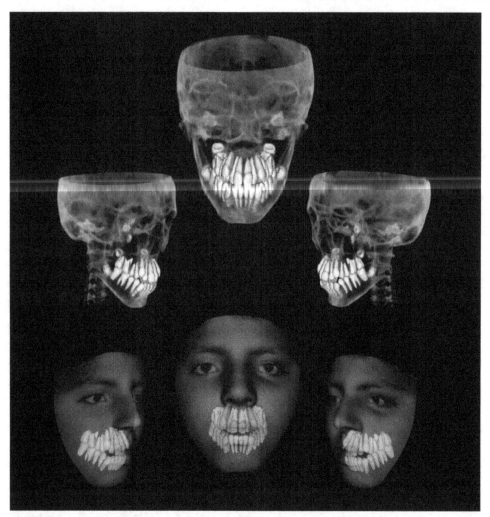

Fig. 7. Dual volume superimposition: the digital model superimposed on a 3D skull volume and a 3D facial photograph provides an excellent tool for treatment simulation and for the evaluation of the anatomical relationships between the teeth, the skeletal, and the soft tissues.

3. Cone beam computed tomography and airway analysis

Airway disorders are a common cause of malocclusions and might result in the classical appearance of adenoid facies. The results of a retrospective review of 500 orthodontic patients showed that 18.2 percent of the patients had airway-related problems. Variations in airway morphology and dimensions are commonly related to hereditary or functional disorders. Despite the cause or the effect, any airway problem has to be properly diagnosed and treated as soon as it is identified. Methods that are traditionally used to assess the airway include cephalometry, rhinoendoscopy, and tomography (Subtenley & Baker, 1965; Fujiki & Rossato, 1999; Filho et al., 2001; Abramson et al., 2010).

Mandibular advancement device, tongue retraining device, and a continous positive airflow pressure appliance are the most common orthodontic therapeutic options for patients with breathing disorders. The assessment of the patient's airway plays a primary role in planning the management strategy, especially in patients suffering from mouth breathing, adenoid hypertrophy, or sleep apnea. The 2D lateral cephalograms offer limited information due to the difficulty in identifying the soft tissue contour in the third dimension thus restricting evaluation of areas and volumes. Currently, there appears to be no better way to assess the airway than by using CBCT imaging (Halazonetis, 2005; Aboudara et al., 2009).

3D CBCT images offer accurate representation of the airway. The CBCT data with the use of different software systems allows better visualization, volumetric measurements, and patency assessment of the airway, as well as the precise distinction between the soft tissues and the airway space. Several studies questioned the reliability of the 3D methods and indicated high reliability and accuracy of area and volume measurements using this technique. Clinicians can more easily perform the volumetric measurements and also calculate the cross-sectional areas of the airway in 3 planes of space: coronal, sagittal, and axial. In addition, the option provided by some softwares for detecting and measuring the most constricted area in the airway provides essential diagnostic clinical information especially in obstructive sleep apnea patients (Ogawa et al., 2007; Aboudara et al., 2009; Abramson et al., 2010) (Figures 8 and 9).

4. 3D cephalometry

Cephalometric analysis in orthodontics is an important diagnostic tool for the assessment of craniofacial morphology. The lateral cephalograms enable orthodontists to determine the size and shape of the jaws, their position in sagittal and vertical relation to the anterior base of the skull, and their position in relation to each other. An analytical method is used to identify and analyze the necessary parameters. It involves determining hard tissue and soft tissue landmarks, and making angular and linear measurements. The information provided by the lateral cephalogram about the vertical and sagittal structure of the facial skull cannot be obtained by any other diagnostic measure. However, cephalometric measurements on the 2D images suffer from several limitations such as the difficulty in locating some reference points and landmarks, image distortion, differences in magnifications, superimposition of the bilateral craniofacial structures, and measurement errors. Another important drawback of lateral and frontal cephalograms is the lack of information about cross-sectional area and volume (Adams et al., 2004; Lenza et al., 2010).

CBCT provide a 3D method for cephalometric analysis (Figure 10). Compared with the traditional cephalometric radiographs, the CBCT produces images that are anatomically true (real-size 1:1 scale) with accurate volumetric 3D depiction of hard and soft tissues of the skull and lack of superimposition of the anatomical structures. Other advantages of this method over the 2D cephalometric analysis include the reduced radiation exposure (as the 3D visualization software generates a 2D lateral image from the 3D data set) and the high precision of the linear and angular measurements obtained. Reliability studies demonstrated that cephalograms reconstructed from CBCT data have no statistically significant differences in linear and angular measurements relative to traditional cephalograms, whereas measurement error from CBCT images are lower than those from cephalograms (Kumar et al., 2007; Moshiri et al., 2007; Kumar et al., 2008).

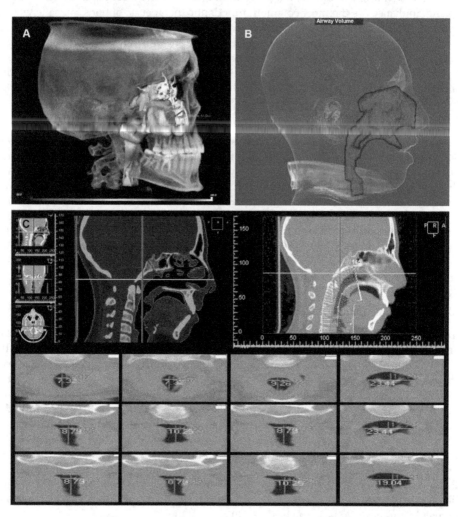

Fig. 8. Volumetric measurements of the airway can be done using different softwares each with a different way of performing the calculations. A) using the InVivoDental software (Anatomage Inc, San Jose, CA), the operator first manually trace the airway passage and then the software will calculate it selectively, B) total airway volume can be calculated by filling in the airway space automatically using the Dolphin software (Dolphin Imaging & Management solutions, Chatsworth, CA), and C) using 3dMD software (3dMD LLC, Atlanta, GA), segmentation for the airway is done first and then the selected areas to be measured will be automatically turned up to a multiple axial slices and the software will calculate the height and width of each slice and give the total airway volume.

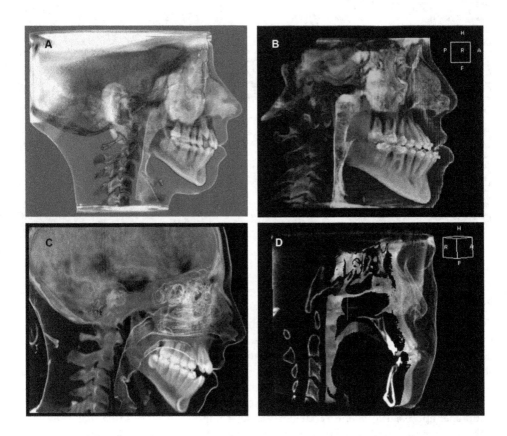

Fig. 9. Volume-rendered CBCT images for the airway in either color enhanced form (A, B, and C) or shaded form (D) where the colors or the shadow are used to aid better visualization and assessment of the airway, as well as correlations with the surrounding head and neck structures. Images generated using the Dolphin software (A), 3dMD (B and D), and InVivoDental (C).

For 3D cephalometry, the anatomical landmarks are identified on 3D surface-rendered volumes or models obtained from CBCT data. In the tracing step, cephalometric planes are defined using either three or four landmarks instead of the two landmarks traditionally used in 2D cephalometry. Beside the elimination of the superimposition of bilateral structures and unequal enlargement artifacts, this also allows for the evaluation of the right and the left sides of the skull independently. The quality and the visibility of the 3D cephalometric landmarks and parameters vary among the different scanners and depend mainly on the scan field of view (FOV) selection, the 3D model segmentation threshold, and image artifacts (Swennen & Schutyser, 2006; Halazonetis, 2005).

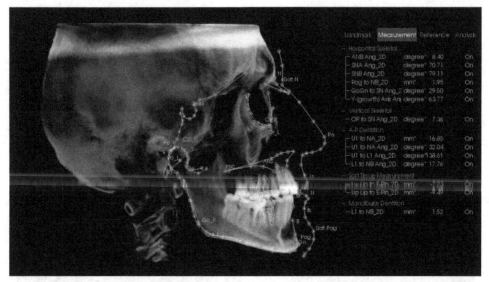

Fig. 10. Linear and angular parameters used for 3D cephalometric analysis (InVivoDental software).

5. 3D superimposition

One of the main advantages of the CBCT is that it allows superimposition of serial images to evaluate the growth and treatment changes. This is an efficient way for showing areas of bone displacement and remodeling, as well as demonstrating the changes in size, shape, and shift in positions of skeletal and soft tissues as a result of either orthodontic or surgical treatments. The 2D cepahalograms have been traditionally used to evaluate these growth or treatment changes based on stable reference structures or anatomical landmarks. The traditional approach to lateral cephalometric superimposition is based on using the most stable anatomical landmarks. For example, the sella turcica for the cranial base registration, the lingual curvature of the palate for the maxillary bony structures, the internal cortical outline of the symphysis, and the mandibular canal for the mandible. However, a major limitation of the 2D representation of a 3D structure with the difficulty in identification of the landmarks is due to the superimposition of multiple structures. In contrast, 3D images provided easier and more accurate anatomical landmark registration (Cevidanes et al., 2005; Lagravere et al., 2006).

The available software tools and options allow optimal alignment of the 3D CBCT datasets at different time points with high precision and accuracy after identification of specific anatomical landmarks and structures. The computed registration is then applied to the segmented structures to measure changes due to orthodontic treatment or surgery. Surface distance calculations are then used for the purpose of accurate quantification of the changes or displacement due to either growth or treatment. Color mapping can show surface area distance differences between two 3D objects or 3D facial photographs (Cevidanes et al., 2005) (Figures 11, 12, and 13).

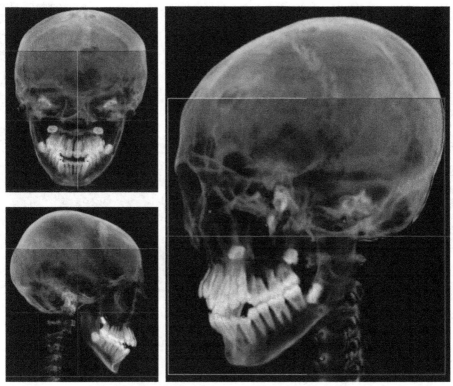

Fig. 11. Demonstration of superimposition of the pre- (brown) and post - (blue) treatment skull models of a 12 years old patient treated with rapid maxillary expansion for a constricted maxillary arch. The use of different colors highlights the changes between the two scans.

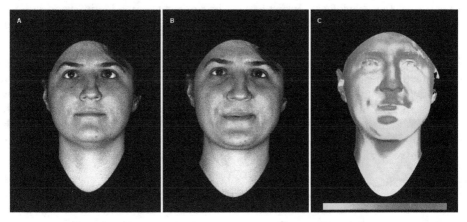

Fig. 12. Three-dimensional facial photograph of a trumpet player: in the rest position (A), during blowing (B), and color mapping (C) used to demonstrate the differences between the two positions.

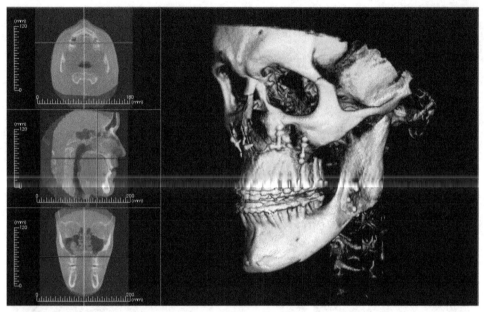

Fig. 13. The changes and shift in position of skeletal structures resulting from orthognathic surgery for correction of mandibular prognathism in 23 years old female patient demonstrated by superimposition of serial 3D images of skull volumes using 2 different color codes.

6. 3D facial photographs

With the introduction of a new system and software, the applicability of 3D photographs in daily orthodontic practice became possible. Photographic soft tissue profile analysis, evaluation of the craniofacial growth and development, orthodontic diagnosis, and measurements of the aesthetic facial parameters can all be professionally performed on these photographs.

One of the gold standard diagnostic tools in orthognathic surgery and preoperative orthodontic treatment is the 2-D facial photographs that consequently reveal limitations in describing the 3D structures of a patient's face. CBCT and the newly introduced imaging techniques such as the 3D stereophotogrammetry (3D photographs) allows exploring the human face 3-dimensionally with multiple useful applications that ranges from using the facial scans to measure all the aesthetic facial parameters to orthodontic diagnosis and evaluation of the craniofacial growth and development (Lane & Harrell, 2008).

Stereophotogrammetry is a method of obtaining an image by means of one or more stereo pairs of photographs being taken simultaneously. The 3D photo camera is used to capture the soft tissue surface of the face with correct geometry and texture information. The technique is based on the triangulation and fringe projection method. Image fusion (i.e., registration of a 3D photograph upon a CBCT) results in an accurate and photorealistic digital 3D data set of a patient's face (Maal et al., 2008).

The registration of pre- and post-operative 3D photographs has many important applications, which mainly include the evaluation of treatment outcomes in orthognathic surgery or orthodontic treatment. After registration or matching of the 3D photographs, the differences between the pre- and post-photographs can be visualized by a color scale or map. In this way, results of the treatment can be evaluated quantitatively and objectively. Other useful applications of comparing different 3D photographs are the evaluation of pathological lesions or swelling such as abscess or tumors over time, cross-sectional growth changes, and the establishment of databases for normative populations. For clinical use, the registration process of pre- and post-treatment 3D photographs has to be very accurate (Metzger et al., 2007; Maal et al., 2010).

One of the recently introduced software features allow the facial photograph to be morphed onto a digital imaging and communications in medicine (DICOM) dataset where the 3D volume can generate a simulated 3D projection of the face in any frontal, lateral, or user-defined view of the face. By changing the translucency of the image, the correlation between the facial soft tissues to the skeleton can be determined. This has great implications in planning orthognathic surgery, orthodontic treatment, or other craniofacial therapies that could affect the facial appearance (Harrell, 2009; Schendel & Lane, 2009) (Figure 14).

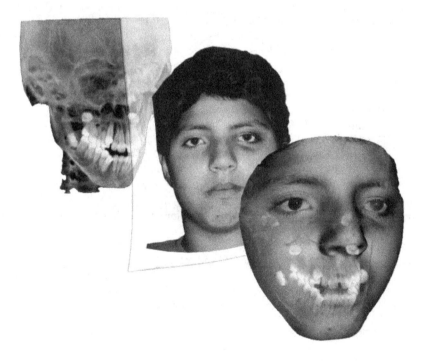

Fig. 14. Facial photographs morphed onto 3D skeletal volume can be used for measurements of the aesthetic facial parameters and soft tissue profile analysis, as well as treatment simulation.

7. Conclusion

CBCT has become widely available and acceptable by the orthodontic community especially as the radiation exposure and cost decreases. The continuous advancements in the imaging machines, techniques, and softwares have added valuable improvement in its diagnostic capabilities. In addition, the ease of image manipulation and its relevancy to the clinical setting offers orthodontists and clinicians the chance for improved diagnosis. Craniofacial imaging is expected to become totally digital in the near future. The orthodontic community needs to increase their knowledge, and evaluate its clinical relevancy and reliability, as well as consider its other applications.

8. References

Aboudara, C., Nielsen, I. & Huang, J. (2009). Comparison of human airway space using conventional lateral headfilms and three-dimensional reconstruction from cone-beam computed tomography. Am J Orthod Dentofac Orthop 135:468-479.

Abramson, Z., Susarla, S., August, M., Troulis, M. & Kaban, L. (2010). Three-dimensional computed tomographic analysis of airway anatomy in patients with obstructive sleep apnea. J Oral Maxillofac Surg 68:354-362.

Adams, G., Gansky, S., Miller, A., Harell, W. & Hatcher D. (2004). Comparison between traditional 2-dimensional cephalometry and a 3-dimensional approach on human dry skull. Am J Orthod Dentofac Orthop 126:397-409.

Cevidanes, L., Bailey, L. & Tucker, GR.(2005). Superimpositon of 3D cone-beam CT models of orthognathic surgery patients. Dentomaxillofac Radiol 34:369-375.

Cevidanes, L., Oliveira, A., Grauer, D., Styner, M. & Proffit, W. (2011). Clinical application of 3D imaging for assessment of treatment outcomes. Semin Orthod 17:72-80.

Dalstra, M. & Melsen, B. (2009). From alginate impressions to virtual digital models. J Orthod 36:36-41.

De Vos, W., Casselman, J. & Swennen, G. (2009). Cone-beam computerized tomography (CBCT) imaging of the oral and maxillofacial region: A systemic review of the literature. Int J Oral Maxillofac Surg 38(6):609-25.

Enciso, R., Memon, A. & Fidaleo, D. (2003). The virtual craniofacial patient: 3D jaw modeling and animation. Stud Health Technol Inform 94:65-71.

Filho, D., Raveli, D., Raveli, R., De Castro, L. & Gandin, L. (2001). A comparison of nasopharyngeal endoscopy and lateral cephalometric radiography in the diagnosis of nasopharyngeal airway obstruction. Am J Orthod Dentofac Orthop 120:348-352.

Fujiki, P. & Rossato, C. (1999). Influencia da hipertrofa adenoideana no crescimento e desenvolvimento craniodentofacial. Ortodontia 32:70-79.

Halazonetis, D. (2005). From 2-dimensional cephalograms to 3-dimensional computed tomography scans. Am J Orthod Dentofac Orthop 127: 627–637

Harrell, W. (2009). 3D diagnosis and treatment planning in orthodontics. Semin Orthod 15:35-41.

Hernandez-Soler, V., Enciso, R. & Cisneros, G. (2011). The virtual patient specific-model and the virtual dental model. Semin Orthod 17:46-48.

Hilgers, M., Scarfe, S. & Scheetz, J. (2005). Accuracy of linear temporomandibular joint measurements with cone beam computed tomography and digital cephalometric radiography. Am J Orthod Dentofacial Orthop 128:803-811.

Honey, O., Scarfe, W. & Hilgers, M. (2007). Accuracy of cone-beam computed tomography imaging of the temporomandibular joint: Comparisons with panoramic radiology and linear tomography. Am J Orthod Dentofacial Orthop 132:429-438.

Huang, J., Bumann, A. & Mah, J. (2005). Three dimensional radiographic analysis in orthodontics. JCO 7:421-428.

Kapila, S., Conley RS. & Harrell, Jr. (2011). The current status of cone beam computed tomography imaging in orthodontics. Dentomaxillofacial Radiology 40:24-34.

Kumar, V., Ludlow, J., Mol, A. & Cevidanes, L. (2007). Comparison of conventional and cone beam CT synthesized cephalograms. Dentomaxillofacial Radiology 36: 263–269

Kumar, V., Ludlow, J., Cevidanes, L. & Mol, A. (2008). In vivo comparison of conventional and cone beam CT synthesized cephalograms. Angle Orthodontist 78: 873–879

Lagravere, M., Hansen, L., Harzer, W. & Major, P. (2006). Plane orientation for standardization in 3-dimensional cephalometric analysis with computerized tomography imaging. Am J Orthod Dentofac Orthop 129:601-4.

Lane, C. & Harrell, W. (2008). Completing the 3-dimensional picture. Am J Orthod Dentofac Orthop 133:612-20.

Lenza, M., Lenza, MM., Dalstra, M., Melsen, B. & Cattaneo, PM. (2010). An analysis of different approaches to the assessment of upper airway morphology: a CBCT study. Orthod Craniofac Res 13:96-105.

Maal, T., Plooij, J., Rangel, F., Mollemans, W., Schutyser, F. & Berge, S. (2008). The accuracy of matching three-dimensional photographs with skin surfaces derived from cone-beam computed tomography. J Oral Maxillofac Surg 37:641-646.

Maal, T., Loon, B., Plooij, J., Rangel, F., Ettema, A., Borstlap, W. & Berge, S. (2010). Registration of 3-dimensional facial photographs for clinical use. J Oral Maxillofac Surg 68:2391-2401.

Mah, J.& Hatcher, D. (2005) Craniofacial imaging in orthodontics. In: Graber, TM., Vanarsdall, RL. & Vig, KWL., editors. Orthodontics, current principles and techniques. 4th ed. St Louis: Mosby.

Mah, J., Yi, L., Huang, R. & Choo, H. (2011). Advanced applications of cone beam computed tomography in orthodontics. Semin Orthod 17:57-71.

Metzger, MC., Hohlweg-Majert, B. & Schon, R. (2007). Verification of clinical precision after computer-aided reconstruction in craniomaxillofacial surgery. Oral Surg Oral Med Oral Pathol Oral Radiol Endod 104:e1.

Molen, A. (2011). Comparing cone beam computed tomography systems from an orthodontic perspective. Semin Orthod 17:34-38.

Moshiri, M., Scarfe, W., Hilgers, M., Scheetz, J., Silveira, A. & Farman, A. (2007). Accuracy of linear measurements from imaging plate and lateral cephalometric images derived from cone-beam computed tomography. Am J Orthod Dentofac Orthop 132: 550–560

Ogawa, T., Enciso, R., Shintaku, W. & Clark, G. (2007). Evaluation of cross-section airway configuration of obstructive sleep apnea. Oral Surg Oral Med Oral Pathol Oral Radiol Endod 103:102-8.

Schendel, S. & Lane, C. (2009). 3D orthognathic surgery simulation using image fusion. Semin Orthod 15:48-56.

Subtelney, J. & Baker, H. (1956). The significance of adenoid tissue in velopharyngeal function. Plastic and Reconstructive Surgery 17:235-250.

Swennen, G. & Schutyser, F. (2006). Three-dimensional cephalometry: spiral multi-slice vs cone-beam computed tomography. Am J Orthod Dentofac Orthop 130: 410–416

Valiathan, A., Dhar, S. & Verma, N. (2008). 3D CT imaging in orthodontics: Adding a new dimension to diagnosis and treatment planning. Trends Biomater Artif Organs 21(2):116-120.

Permissions

The contributors of this book come from diverse backgrounds, making this book a truly international effort. This book will bring forth new frontiers with its revolutionizing research information and detailed analysis of the nascent developments around the world.

We would like to thank Farid Bourzgui, for lending his expertise to make the book truly unique. He has played a crucial role in the development of this book. Without his invaluable contribution this book wouldn't have been possible. He has made vital efforts to compile up to date information on the varied aspects of this subject to make this book a valuable addition to the collection of many professionals and students.

This book was conceptualized with the vision of imparting up-to-date information and advanced data in this field. To ensure the same, a matchless editorial board was set up. Every individual on the board went through rigorous rounds of assessment to prove their worth. After which they invested a large part of their time researching and compiling the most relevant data for our readers. Conferences and sessions were held from time to time between the editorial board and the contributing authors to present the data in the most comprehensible form. The editorial team has worked tirelessly to provide valuable and valid information to help people across the globe.

Every chapter published in this book has been scrutinized by our experts. Their significance has been extensively debated. The topics covered herein carry significant findings which will fuel the growth of the discipline. They may even be implemented as practical applications or may be referred to as a beginning point for another development. Chapters in this book were first published by InTech; hereby published with permission under the Creative Commons Attribution License or equivalent.

The editorial board has been involved in producing this book since its inception. They have spent rigorous hours researching and exploring the diverse topics which have resulted in the successful publishing of this book. They have passed on their knowledge of decades through this book. To expedite this challenging task, the publisher supported the team at every step. A small team of assistant editors was also appointed to further simplify the editing procedure and attain best results for the readers.

Our editorial team has been hand-picked from every corner of the world. Their multi-ethnicity adds dynamic inputs to the discussions which result in innovative outcomes. These outcomes are then further discussed with the researchers and contributors who give their valuable feedback and opinion regarding the same. The feedback is then collaborated with the researches and they are edited in a comprehensive manner to aid the understanding of the subject.

Apart from the editorial board, the designing team has also invested a significant amount of their time in understanding the subject and creating the most relevant covers. They scrutinized every image to scout for the most suitable representation of the subject and create an appropriate cover for the book.

The publishing team has been involved in this book since its early stages. They were actively engaged in every process, be it collecting the data, connecting with the contributors or procuring relevant information. The team has been an ardent support to the editorial, designing and production team. Their endless efforts to recruit the best for this project, has resulted in the accomplishment of this book. They are a veteran in the field of academics and their pool of knowledge is as vast as their experience in printing. Their expertise and guidance has proved useful at every step. Their uncompromising quality standards have made this book an exceptional effort. Their encouragement from time to time has been an inspiration for everyone.

The publisher and the editorial board hope that this book will prove to be a valuable piece of knowledge for researchers, students, practitioners and scholars across the globe.

List of Contributors

Carlos Bellot-Arcís, José María Montiel-Company and José Manuel Almerich-Silla
Stomatology Department, University of Valencia, Spain

C. Jiménez-Caro, F. de Carlos and J. Cobo
Instituto Asturiano de Odontología, Oviedo, Spain
Departamento de Cirugía y Especialidades, Médico-Quirúrgicas (sección de Odontología), Universidad de Oviedo, Spain

A.A. Suárez
Instituto Asturiano de Odontología, Oviedo, Spain
Departamento de Construcción e Ingeniería de la, Fabricación (Sección de Ingeniería Mecánica), Universidad de Oviedo, Spain

J.A. Vega
Departamento de Morfología y Biología Celular, Universidad de Oviedo, Spain

Melinda Madléna
Semmelweis University, Hungary

R.A. Al-Sanea
Department of Dentistry-Central Region, National Guards Health Affairs, Kingdom of Saudi Arabia

B. Kusnoto and C.A. Evans
Department of Orthodontics, University of Illinois at Chicago, USA

Seung-Ho Ohk
Department of Oral Microbiology, Korea

Hyeon-Shik Hwang
Department of Orthodontics and Dental Science, Research Institute, Chonnam National University, Korea

Gladia Toledo Mayarí
School of Dentistry/ Havana Medical University, Cuba

Liliana M. Otero
University of Kentucky, USA
Pontificia Universidad Javeriana, Colombia

James K. Hartsfield Jr. and Lorri Ann Morford
University of Kentucky, USA

Eman Allam, Katherine Kula and L. Jack Windsor
Indiana University School of Dentistry, Indianapolis, USA

Ahmed Ghoneima
Indiana University School of Dentistry, Indianapolis, USA
Faculty of Dental Medicine, Al-Azhar University, Cairo, Egypt